D1029552

The Exercising Adult

The Exercising Adult

edited by
Robert C. Cantu, M.D.

Chairman, Department of Surgery
Chief, Neurosurgical Service
Director, Service of Sports Medicine
Emerson Hospital
Concord, Massachusetts

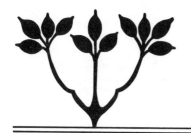

THE COLLAMORE PRESS
D.C. Heath and Company
Lexington, Massachusetts
Toronto

Published simultaneously in Canada and the United Kingdom

Printed in the United States of America

International Standard Book Number: 0-669-04509-8

Library of Congress Catalog Card Number: 81-065129

Library of Congress Cataloging in Publication Data
Main entry under title:

The Exercising Adult.

   Papers presented at the annual meeting of the New England Chapter of the American College of Sports Medicine, Nov. 21 and 22, 1980.
   Includes index.
   1. Sports medicine—Congresses. 2. Exercise—Physiological aspects—Congresses. 3. Cardiacs—Rehabilitation—Congresses. 4. Physical fitness—Congresses. I. Cantu, Robert C. II. American College of Sports Medicine. New England Chapter.
RC1201.E93   613.7'1   81-65129
ISBN 0-669-04509-8   AACR2

Contents

Foreword

More and more Americans are becoming active in sports and physical fitness. In a sense, exercise is the miracle drug of our time. It enhances the natural, miraculous ways in which our bodies protect us from disease. It can have a vital role in rehabilitation from injury or illness. Physical fitness is also related to one's mental well-being. Running, for example, has been used effectively to treat certain mental conditions, such as depression.

Experts in sports medicine are encouraged by the renewed interest in fitness. It is a popular movement that public officials and medical professionals ought to strengthen. Exercise is a vital element of preventive and rehabilitative health. Speaking as an early morning runner myself, I can assert that exercise can even be fun.

The good news on sports and fitness is that it is part of a broader movement. Government and the medical profession are putting increased emphasis on preventing illness and injury. We still spend too little on prevention, relative to treatment.

Federal spending on health enters a new era in 1981. I cannot predict the fate of current health programs under a new administration and a more conservative Congress. President Reagan has promised to boost military spending, cut taxes, and balance the budget. His fudge factor is all the waste to be cut from the budget. The sad irony is that such cuts tend to be false economies. When dollars are scarce, it becomes particularly important to invest them in effective programs to prevent future costs that are far more expensive. As health spending faces tougher competition for federal dollars, preventive approaches must be emphasized even more strongly.

Health Promotion

One investment in preventive health is federal support for health-maintenance organizations. Federal spending for such organizations totaled $54 million in fiscal 1980. For the year that began October 1, 1981 the level is projected to increase to $62 million. Continued expansion of this program is important.

Another recent, positive development is the Office of Health Promotion. It has set up the National Health Information Clearinghouse. In January 1981, the office began an ambitious media campaign centered on a healthstyle test. This is a short self-test to rate personal health habits. The healthstyle project addresses a basic reality: personal lifestyle choices are a major factor in illness, injury, and death. Ultimately, neither Uncle Sam nor Doctor Smith can make individuals stop smoking, overeating, atrophying, or drunk-driving. But more and better information must be provided to promote good health.

Consider young women. Washington has made their opportunities for school sports participation far more equal in recent years. This can be expected to have a positive health impact. At the same time, the proportion of teen-age girls who smoke has been rising. Clever cigarette ads emphasize sophistication, independence, and sexual equality, but the bottom line is that these young women will have a more equal chance for cancer, emphysema, and heart disease in the twenty-first century. The 1979 surgeon general's *Report on Smoking and Health* emphasized the dangers of smoking to women. Clearly, health promotion requires far more than facts about health dangers. If health promotion is to fight Madison Avenue, it has to use equivalent tools. The professionalism that sells tar and nicotine as liberation can also be used to sell better health.

Research is increasing our knowledge of how to make health messages compelling. The message and the method have to be sensitive to social milieu. In the case of teen-age smoking, for example, long-range health dangers are overcome by peer pressure and posturing. Dr. Alfred McAlister of Harvard's School of Public Health has had positive results by training early teens to be ready with a thoughtful reaction to pressures to smoke.

Another mechanism is the almighty dollar—private dollars. Analysis & Computer Systems Inc. in Bedford, Massachusetts, gives workers $1,000 if they quit smoking and $10 for every pound they lose. Such programs, which are multiplying, pay off in fewer sick days, better morale, lower turnover, and higher productivity overall. They may also result in lower health-insurance premiums.

A health milestone was reached in 1980 with release of the first surgeon general's report on health promotion and disease prevention, entitled *Healthy People*. The report reminded us all that we have come to take the cures of modern medicine almost for granted. One forgets that Americans' current health is due more to preventing disease than from curing it after it strikes. The preventive means were better sanitation and nutrition and effective immunizations.

The surgeon general's report chose fifteen priority action areas—such as family planning, toxic agents, and nutrition—where action is vital to prolong life expectancies. It lists measurable health goals for the 1980s. The surgeon general called for a partnership of committed individuals, communities, employers, voluntary agencies, and health professionals. His proposals could lead to major gains in the health of Americans.

Internationally, a great deal of research is being aimed at health promotion among youth. Young people may become much more of a target of long-term strategies for preventing illness and injury. It may be much easier (and cheaper) to dissuade teen-agers from starting smoking than to help mature adults get unhooked. We should help all age groups but put federal dollars where they will be the most effective.

There are other reasons to emphasize young people. By definition, they have the most potential years to lose by fatal illness. There is an equity issue too. We do not expect children and teen-agers to be as knowledgeable and responsible as adults. We are obligated to foster healthful attitudes and practices among our youth.

Public policy-makers and medical professionals must improve health promotion aimed at our youth. In addition to cigarette smoking, other major prevention issues involving prevention focus on young Americans.

Family Planning. Of more than 4 million pregnancies a year, 1 million are terminated by legal abortion. Another estimated 1 million are unplanned.

Sexually Transmitted Diseases. There were 10 million cases in 1977, 86% between the ages of 15 and 29. That is simply unacceptable.

Driving and Drinking. Teen-agers and young adults have the highest highway death rate. One-third of all fatalities are between 15 and 24 years old. At least half of all traffic deaths are alcohol-related. Current efforts are not good enough. We are used to these statistics; otherwise, this traffic-death rate would be considered an epidemic...the lethal equivalent of war.

Health and Limits

In 1980 Americans spent over $200 billion on health. In 1984 it is projected that $400 billion will be spent. Obviously, such an escalation in health spending may be hazardous to the health of our economy. We face fiscal limits and hard choices, but scarce dollars make preventive approaches all the more essential.

There are two other kinds of limits that can affect human health drastically: finite energy resources and environmental limits. Regarding energy, we are still being cavalier about our economic security and survival itself. The survival instinct is supposed to be very strong, but as a society we have not shown it. If suddenly we faced fuel oil shortages this winter, the health cost could include elderly and ill citizens freezing to death in their homes, and if we think the federal health budget is about to be stretched tight, we can imagine the disaster in a depression triggered by a new OPEC oil embargo.

We are drifting into biosphere overload of the environment. Just as many people abuse the regenerative balance of their own bodies, we have exploited and endangered the entire biosphere. I have chaired hearings on two dangers related to coal—acid rain and the potential greenhouse effect. Acid rain, which is associated with respiratory ailments, is killing lakes and entering the food chain. The possible greenhouse effect in the next century might create drastic climatic changes, including the submersion of coastal areas.

The Senate has been unable to legislate on another major environmental issue: money to clean up toxic waste accumulations like that at Love Canal. Under the pending bill, the industry would underwrite 75% of the cleanup fund through a special tax at the production level. The U.S. Treasury would pay the rest.

Conclusion

Collectively, we have great experience and expertise in rehabilitation, and our skills can nurture the natural healing process of someone injured or severely disabled. Sports and fitness may be more crucial to a disabled person than to someone more able-bodied. Exercise can improve mobility and strength and may reduce depression. Rehabilitative work is personally satisfying. Moreover, some recent, dramatic, technological advances in rehabilitation services have been achieved. For example, the remarkable progress in research on spinal cord injuries is very encouraging.

Dedicated individuals can be helped to make their own miracles, beat disabilities, and reach their human maximum. In contrast to them are so many others who enable their health to weaken because of laziness, conformity, or ignorance of consequences. The dormant majority who fritter away their health (for whatever reason) constitute a society that is disabling itself. We must work together to devise lean, innovative, effective programs to rehabilitate and promote the health of Americans as a whole.

Finally, perhaps we could rededicate ourselves to the health of American society in the memory of a man who embodied it. He was filled with life, with vigor, as if it might all be gone too soon. He stood for maximizing human potential. President Kennedy died 17 years ago, but he left his spirit in many places and in many people. It is in the President's Council on Physical Fitness and Sports. It is in the Peace Corps, which shaped my own life more than any other experience. I hope it is in all of us. Let us work together to help Americans fill their lives with fitness and health.

Senator Paul E. Tsongas

Preface

As the 1980s begin, those in sports medicine must accept the challenge to educate the nation's coaches, trainers, physical therapists, nutritionists, exercise specialists, paramedical personnel, competitive and recreational athletes, and nonathletic lay persons. The task is to apply pure knowledge to the practical problems of improving performance and the quality of life, while simultaneously avoiding injury. Many myths and half-truths have been propagated by the media, athletes, lay persons, paramedics, and even some physicians, all without a proper exercise physiology background. These half-truths must be replaced with sound facts.

The decade of the 1970s brought a fitness boom as the public began to realize that the three major killers—heart disease, cancer, and diabetes—are largely the result of an inappropriate lifestyle (inactivity and obesity) and self-pollution (smoking, alcohol, and drug abuse). The words of the late Dr. John Knowles of the Rockefeller Foundation were heeded: "The next major advance in the health of the American people will result only from what the individual is willing to do for himself."

The response was, indeed, dramatic as millions of Americans engaged in a fitness mania with the tennis boom giving way to a tidal wave of jogging and running. While basically positive, this often excessively overenthusiastic, usually underinformed headlong dash into fitness has many potential hazards. Deaths were attributed both to extreme fad diets and too rapidly pursuing vigorous exercise regimens. Sports medicine services sprang up in many hospitals to treat the flood of overuse musculoskeletal injuries so prevalent in the recreational athlete.

Sports medicine is involved not only with the prevention and treatment of injuries but equally with the promotion of health and fitness through aerobic exercise, appropriate lifestyles, and adequate nutrition. Newer subdivisions include cardiac rehabilitation, sports psychology, and biomechanics in addition to the more basic sports physiology and nutrition.

Those in sports medicine believe the greatest present potential for improving one's health is to be realized in what one does and does not do to oneself. Individual decisions about diet, exercise, and smoking are critical. A recent study at Massachusetts General Hospital disclosed that three out of five hospitalizations could have been avoided if people had taken better care of themselves. While exercise alone is no panacea, the medical evidence is overwhelming that people who live sensibly and keep fit are healthier, feel better, are more productive, have lower absenteeism and better morale at work, and live longer.

A new direction concentrating on positive health rather than curative treatment must be undertaken. Health cannot be given or brought to the

American people; they must learn to take better care of themselves in order to avoid illness and to function at full capacity. Health depends less on medicine than on genetics, lifestyle, environment, and cultural factors. People must learn how to help themselves not to require medical attention. The U.S. government realizes that the most potent tool to limit health-care expenditures is to concentrate on keeping people healthy rather than returning them to health after they have become ill.

This book is devoted to exposing the many myths and presenting the unblemished facts in the areas of exercise testing, the latest fitness programs, exercise and cardiac rehabilitation, diabetes, gerontology, nutrition, psychology, and sports injuries. The burning desire behind this book is to afford the exercising adult the maximal opportunity for positive health maintenance.

The five parts of this book span all three areas of sports medicine: trauma, medicine, and research. In the first part, Drs. Michael D. Klein and Donald A. Weiner discuss the use of exercise testing to safely outline an exercise program for the adult. Current controversies are fully examined. Dr. Michael Sachs, in this same section, presents the latest psychological research on the subject of compliance and addiction to exercise. Those factors that mitigate for and against successfully following an exercise program are elucidated.

The second part is devoted to describing a number of different exercise programs currently being marketed by industry and academic institutions as well as commercial-for-profit companies. Here the exercising adult has a wide array of exercise regimens from which one may adapt either an entire routine or parts from several to compose one's own unique exercise program. A thorough explanation of the requirements (composition, duration, intensity, frequency) of an adequate fitness program depending on one's current state of fitness and objectives is especially well outlined by Drs. Thomas Manfredi and W. Jay Gillespie.

Special considerations for the exercising adult are covered in the third part. Nutrition, a multibillion dollar industry rampant with hype and quackery, is put into sharp perspective regarding the special needs of the vigorously exercising adult. A clear distinction is made between scientific fact and unproven theory. All exercising adults will find this section essential to thoughtfully planning their own nutrition to maximize health and performance.

For those who either personally have diabetes or have family or friends afflicted with this third leading cause of death in the United States, the chapter by Dr. Lee N. Cunningham, a research associate of the Joslin Clinic, is vital. This chapter discusses the special concerns and benefits exercise poses for the diabetic from diet to hypoglycemic reactions to foot care.

Section four, devoted to cardiac rehabilitation, examines and cites examples of the different types of inpatient and outpatient cardiac rehabilitation programs. Since coronary artery disease is the leading cause of death in the United States, cardiac rehabilitation programs are of major medical importance.

The final part, sports injuries, deals with an area of sports medicine where major advances are being made in both prevention and treatment. Dr. Arthur L. Boland, head surgeon, Harvard Athletic Department, and Dr. Lyle J. Micheli, director, Division of Sports Medicine, Children's Hospital Medical Center, Boston, discuss upper- and lower-extremity injuries respectively. Head and spine injuries are covered in my chapters, chapters 14 and 15. All three of us bring to our respective areas not only the medical expertise of our surgical training and experience but also that gleaned from having been collegiate and now recreational athletes and team physicians. Through this combined experience emerges the realization that the prevention of sports injuries is a responsibility shared by coaches, trainers, and team physicians with the athlete.

The athlete, as student or professional, must heed the words of Machiavelli: "Fortune is the arbiter of half the things we do, leaving the other half or so to be controlled by ourselves." Those in sports medicine must forever realize that the major goal is not just the treatment of sports injuries but rather the determination of risk and, thereby, reduction of both the incidence and severity of injuries in sports.

Acknowledgments

This book contains the presentations given at the annual meeting of the New England chapter of the American College of Sports Medicine November 21 and 22, 1980.

I would first like to express my sincere appreciation to Senator Paul E. Tsongas who wrote the foreword; to the many contributing authors who forwarded their excellent manuscripts on schedule, thus enabling this effort to be timely; and to Drs. Lyle J. Micheli and W. Jay Gillespie, the president and president-elect of the New England chapter of the American College of Sports Medicine. I also wish to thank Elizabeth Eagan-Bengston, M.S., Cardiovascular Health and Exercise Center, Northeastern University, and Daria J. Christensen, Division of Sports Medicine, Children's Hospital Medical Center, the annual meeting program coordinators. I also wish to acknowledge the efforts of Bernice McPhee, director of education and training at Emerson Hospital, who coordinated the taping of this meeting. Finally, a special word of thanks to my secretary Pat Blackey for her skill in typing this manuscript while pleasantly and efficiently keeping a busy neurosurgical office running smoothly.

Contributing Authors

Arthur L. Boland, M.D.
Instructor, Orthopaedic Surgery, Harvard Medical School
Chief of Orthopaedics, Harvard University Health Services
Head Surgeon, Harvard Athletic Department
Staff Orthopaedic Surgeon, New England Baptist Hospital
Boston, Massachusetts

David Camaione, Ph.D.
Director, American Cardio-Fitness Center
The University of Connecticut
Hartford, Connecticut

Robert C. Cantu, M.D.
Chief, Neurosurgical Service
Chairman, Department of Surgery
Director, Service of Sports Medicine
Emerson Hospital
Concord, Massachusetts

Catherine Certo, R.P.T., M.S.
Assistant Professor of Physical Therapy
Coordinator, Cardiac Rehabilitation Program
Cardiovascular Health and Exercise Center
Northeastern University
Boston, Massachusetts

Christopher T. Coughlin, M.S.
Exercise Specialist
New England Heart Center
Brookline, Massachusetts

Lee N. Cunningham, D.P.E.
Research Associate, Joslin Clinic
Boston, Massachusetts
Physical Education Department, Fitchburg State College
Fitchburg, Massachusetts

Richard G. Day
Fitness Director, Sentry Insurance Company
Concord, Massachusetts

Nancy V. Dolan, R.N., M.S.N.
Cardiac Rehabilitation Nurse Specialist
New England Heart Center

W. Jay Gillespie, Ed.D.
Associate Professor of Physical Education
Director, Cardiovascular Health and Exercise Center
Northeastern University
Boston, Massachusetts

Gail Handysides, R.N., M.S.N.
Cardiac Clinical Specialist
Coordinator, Cardiac Rehabilitation Program
New England Memorial Hospital
Stoneham, Massachusetts

Michael D. Klein, M.D.
Associate Professor of Medicine, Boston University School of Medicine
Head of Coronary Care, Department of Cardiology,
Boston University Hospital
Medical Director, Cardiovascular Health and Exercise Center,
Northeastern University
Boston, Massachusetts

Gary Klencheski, M.S.
Director and Vice President, Boston Fitcorp
Boston, Massachusetts

Thomas Manfredi, Ph.D.
Chairman of Men's Physical Education
Southern Connecticut State University
New Haven, Connecticut

Lyle J. Micheli, M.D.
Clinical Instructor, Orthopaedic Surgery, Harvard Medical School
Associate Orthopaedic Surgeon
Director, Division of Sports Medicine, Children's Hospital Medical
Center
Boston, Massachusetts

National Dairy Council

Michael L. Sachs, Ph.D.
Department des Sciences de L'Activité Physique
Université du Québec à Trois-Rivières

Donald A. Weiner, M.D.
Director, Exercise Laboratory
Department of Cardiology, Boston University Hospital
Boston University School of Medicine
Boston, Massachusetts

Medical, Physiologic, and Psychologic Assessment Prior to Exercise Training

1

Exercise Testing During a Cardiovascular Fitness Program: Assessment of Cardiac Arrhythmias in a Noncoronary Disease Population

Michael D. Klein, M.D.

There is much information on the use of treadmill exercise testing in the diagnosis of coronary heart disease. The accuracy of this technique, as determined from its sensitivity, specificity, and ability to stratify severity of coronary artery disease has been reviewed elsewhere in this book (see chapter 2). Less information is available on the usefulness of treadmill exercise testing in characterizing rhythm disturbances of the heart. The following report describes the clinical correlates of 338 apparently healthy individuals who underwent treadmill testing as part of a screening procedure prior to entering a cardiovascular fitness program. Special attention was given to 37 individuals who exhibited some form of atrial or ventricular dysrhythmia immediately prior to, during, or in the ten minutes subsequent to completion of a graded treadmill exercise test. Analysis of the data suggested that, in the absence of coronary artery disease, the emergence of atrial and ventricular ectopic activity during treadmill testing correlated either with mitral valve prolapse, hypertension, or primary cardiac arrhythmia.

Methods

The study population was composed of 338 adults, aged 22 to 64 years (39.4 ± 12.8 SD), of which 274 were men, and 64 were women. All were apparently healthy. None had documented heart disease. The presence of a past history of a heart murmur, nonanginal chest pains, palpitations or rapid heart beating, dizzy spells, unusual or unexplained fatigue, or sensitivity of the hands or feet upon exposure to cold was obtained from a standard questionnaire.

Cardiac examination was performed in the supine, sitting, standing,

From The Cardiovascular Health and Exercise Center, Boston-Bouvé College, Northeastern University.

and squatting positions. The valsalva maneuver was carried out in the standing position. Abrupt squatting upon release of the valsalva strain phase was also routinely employed to provide a maximal stimulus for slowing of the heart rate after it had been accelerated during phase three of the valsalva maneuver. Special attention was given to the emergence of systolic clicks or murmurs during any of these maneuvers.

The resting recumbent ECG was reviewed for minor ST-T-wave abnormalities, especially in the inferior and lateral leads, extra systoles, and the presence of delta waves. PR intervals were divided into three categories: less than 0.12 seconds, 0.12 to 0.14 seconds, greater than 0.14 seconds. This classification was adopted because of the known association of Wolff-Parkinson-White syndrome with short PR intervals and episodic reentrant extrasystoles and tachycardias [8], and because of the association of the Lown-Ganong-Levine syndrome with PR intervals of 0.14 seconds or less and supraventricular tachyarrhythmias and atrial premature beats [5].

Prior to treadmill testing, hyperventilation was performed in the sitting position. Rapid breathing was sustained for 15 seconds. The ECG was then repeated in the sitting position and reviewed for new or exaggerated ST-T-wave abnormalities in the inferolateral leads. The Bruce protocol was followed during treadmill testing on a Quintron treadmill. A 12-lead ECG was recorded during each stage on a three channel Hewlett-Packard ECG machine. Additional ECG strips were recorded if extrasystoles occurred at any time during exercise. Repeat 12-lead ECG sequences were taken during a recovery period of 6 to 12 minutes while the subject was walking slowly on the treadmill after it had been returned to ground level.

Results

Ventricular Arrhythmias

Ventricular arrhythmias were recorded in 28 individuals, 17 men and 11 women. In 6 cases, ventricular premature beats (VPB) were observed prior to exercise testing, in 2 instances during exercise testing, in 13 subsequent to treadmill exertion, and in 7 both before and after treadmill exercise. Three individuals exhibited VPB couplet, and in one, a VPB triplet was recorded during submaximal exercise. In no case did ischemic ST changes occur during treadmill testing. One of the men had high voltage on the resting ECG, and another male had borderline low serum potassium. In two men, systolic pressure exceeded 200 mm Hg during treadmill testing.

Of the 11 women with VPB, 9 had evidence of a mitral systolic click, murmur, or both on auscultation. Of these 9, 7 had inferolateral ST straightening on the resting ECG, and 5 showed posthyperventilation T inversion in the inferior or lateral leads. All 7 of these women gave a history of palpitations or dizzy spells. Four acknowledged unusual cold sensitivity in the hands, suggestive of Raynaud phenomenon. Two had occasional non-anginal left-sided chest pains. Three indicated periods of fatigue not related to menstrual periods.

Of the 17 men with VPB, only 2 had evidence of a mitral systolic click, and 1 of these had a provocable mitral systolic murmur as well. One of these 2 males had inferolateral ST straightening and a PR interval of less than 0.14 seconds. Neither, however, showed posthyperventilation T-wave changes. Two men indicated a history of palpitations or dizzy spells. One had unusual cold sensitivity of the hands and feet. None indicated unusual chest pains or fatigue, however.

Atrial Arrhythmias

Atrial premature beats (APB) were recorded in 11 people, nine women and two men. In 3, the APB were recorded before treadmill testing, in 2 during treadmill testing, and in 4 after treadmill exercise. An unusual pattern of ST depression was observed in 2 cases (1 man, 1 woman) only late in the recovery phase, two to three minutes after exercise but was not accompanied by chest pain (see figure 1-1). Three of the nine women had inferolateral ST straightening on the resting ECG and showed inferior or lateral T-wave depression or flattening with hyperventilation. Five of the women

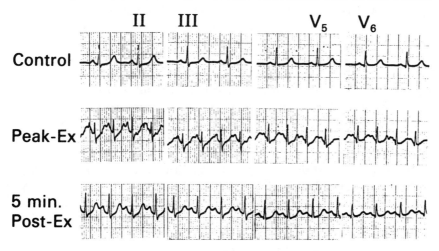

Figure 1-1. 12 Lead ECG

had PR intervals of 0.12 to 0.14 seconds on their resting ECG.

Of the nine women with APB, seven gave a history of palpitations of either skipped beats or paroxysmal tachycardia or dizzy spells. Six of these had occasional left-sided chest pains. Six also indicated a painful sensitivity of the fingers to cold. Four women reported unusual bouts of fatigue not related to menstrual periods.

Of the two men with APB, one gave a history of palpitations, consisting of skipped beats. Neither, however, recalled unusual chest pains, periods of fatigue, or cold sensitivity of the hands. All nine of the women and one of the two men manifested a mitral systolic click or murmur or both during detailed cardiac auscultation.

Discussion

Ventricular premature beats (VPB) can occur during treadmill exercise testing in patients with coronary heart disease. Most likely, they originate in ischemic and partially depolarized myocardium with altered automaticity and conduction, resulting in ectopic or reentrant VPB.

In the present study, 8% (28/338) of apparently healthy people being screened for an adult fitness program exhibited VPB during treadmill testing: 61% were men; 39% were women. In 82% (9/11) of the women evidence for mitral valve prolapse was found on auscultation with a mitral systolic click or murmur or both. A large majority of this group, 78% (7/9), had ST-T abnormalities in the inferolateral leads on the resting ECG, and five showed additional T-wave inversion in some of these leads following hyperventilation [5]. Only 12% (2/17) of the men had auscultatory evidence of mitral valve prolapse, and no consistent inferolateral ECG abnormalities were found in this small group.

A majority of the women (64%) (7/11) gave a history of palpitations in the form of skipped beats. Periodic dizzy spells suggestive of postural hypotension were also noted. Atypical (nonanginal) left-sided chest pains, spells of fatigue, and cold sensitivity were frequently noted by these women. Only 12% (2/17) of the men with VPB indicated a past history of chest pain, and none of these indicated bouts of unusual chest pain, fatigue, or cold sensitivity in their histories.

In 3% (11/338) of the study population, atrial premature beats (APB) were seen during treadmill testing; 82% (9/11) of this group were women. A third of the women had inferolateral ST straightening on the resting ECG and posthyperventilation T inversions in some of these leads. All of the women and one of two men manifested signs of mitral valve prolapse on auscultation—a systolic murmur or click or both.

In 78% (7/9) of the women with APB, there was a history of palpitations consisting of skipped beats or paroxysmal rapid heart action. A majority of this group (6/7) also had left-sided chest pains and cold sensitivity in the hands.

The present data suggest that a majority of people who have APB or VPB during treadmill exercise testing and who do not have coronary heart disease probably have mitral valve prolapse. The majority of these individuals are women, which is in keeping with the known prevalence of this syndrome [7]. Most will have a systolic murmur and click audible at the left sternal border [6]. However, careful auscultation utilizing valsalva and squatting maneuvers or both in tandem may be necessary to evoke these auscultatory events.

Minor repolarization wave abnormalities consisting of ST straightening in the inferolateral leads were often present in both the men and women who had APB or VPB, as noted previously [2]. T-wave inversions often appeared following hyperventilation in some of these leads.

Certain features of the health history pointed toward the likelihood of mitral valve prolapse and APB or VPB with treadmill testing. These included unusual left-sided pains, inexplicable bouts of fatigue, palpitations in the form of skipped beats or tachycardia, cold sensitivity of the hands, postural dizziness. These last two features are suggestive of an unusual autonomic nervous system responsiveness and are consistent with reports of decreased parasympathetic restraint and increased alpha and beta adrenergic responsiveness in women with mitral valve prolapse [3]. Such an altered autonomic control over the circulatory system might also have explained the relatively slow return of heart rate to baseline levels following completion of treadmill exercise observed in several of the patients.

In the few patients with repetitive VPB during treadmill testing, auscultatory evidence of mitral valve prolapse was not heard. Presumably, these individuals had a primary electrical abnormality of the heart, possibly a concealed bypass tract which would permit a recirculation of the electrical wavefront from ventricle to atrial and back again [4].

If isolated APB or VPB with ischemic ST changes arise during treadmill screening for cardiovascular fitness programs, strong consideration should be given to the possibility that these individuals have mitral valve prolapse. Since many of these individuals will have an altered autonomic control over their circulation with evidence for a heightened adrenergic state [1], goals for conditioning their heart rate response to repetitive exercise may not have to be set at a modest level. An understanding of these facts by both exercise instructors and participants in fitness programs is essential if realistic goals are to be achieved and unrealistic fears avoided.

References

1. Boudoulas, H., Reynolds, J.C., Mazzaferri, E., and Wooley, C.F. Metabolic studies in mitral valve prolapse syndrome. *Circulation* 61:1200–1205, 1980.

2. Devereux, R.B., Perloff, J.K., Reichek, N., et al. Mitral valve prolapse. *Circulation* 53:3–14, 1976.

3. Gaffney, F.A., Karlsson, E.S., Campbell, W. et al. Autonomic dysfunction in women with mitral valve prolapse syndrome. *Circulation* 59:894–901, 1979.

4. Josephson, M.E., Horowitz, L.N., and Kastor, J.A. Paroxysmal supraventricular tachycardia in patients wtih mitral valve prolapse. *Circulation* 57:111–115, 1978.

5. Lown, B., Ganong, W.F., and Levine, S.A. Syndrome of short PR interval, normal QRS complex and paroxysmal rapid heart action. *Circulation* 5:693–706, 1952.

6. Markiewicz, W., Stones, J., London, E., et al. Mitral valve prolapse in one hundred presumably healthy young females. *Circulation* 53:464–473, 1976.

7. Procacci, P.M., Savran, S.V., Schreiber, S.L., et al. Prevalence of clinical mitral valve prolapse in 1,169 young women. *N. Engl. J. Med.* 294:1086–1088, 1976.

8. Wolff, L., and White, P.D. Syndrome of short PR interval with abnormal QRS complexes and paroxysmal tachycardia. *Arch. Int. Med.* 28:446–451, 1948.

2 Controversies in Exercise Testing

Donald A. Weiner, M.D.

The medical screening of patients before an exercise program usually consists of taking a detailed history and making a complete physical examination. This approach usually allows the physician to detect overt signs or symptoms of valvular heart disease or congenital heart disease which would limit an exercise program. However, many cases of atherosclerotic coronary artery disease are clinically silent and manifest no signs by physical examination. Thus many physicians will order a noninvasive test to screen for latent coronary artery disease. This usually involves a rest and exercise electrocardiogram which can be used to measure a patient's exercise capacity and to screen for abnormalities on the electrocardiogram which might indicate the presence of coronary artery disease. Although there may be many abnormalities in the electrocardiographic response to exercise such as ventricular arrhythmias, bundle branch blocks, and T-wave abnormalities, changes in the ST-segment response alone appear to be most predictive of the presence of coronary artery disease. Initial studies correlating the results of the exercise test and coronary arteriography demonstrate that in symptomatic men the presence of an abnormal ST-segment response to stress almost always correctly predicts the presence of significant coronary artery disease [1,20,26]. However, similar studies in women [7,30] or asymptomatic men [3,13] suggest that no such correlation exists, which raises questions concerning the test's reliability. This chapter will outline the validity of exercise testing for screening asymptomatic individuals for latent coronary artery disease prior to an exercise program.

Pathophysiology of Stress Testing

The major function of stress testing is to determine whether the coronary circulation can increase oxygen supply to the myocardium in response to the increased myocardial oxygen demands caused by exercise. This is best and most safely accomplished by using isotonic or dynamic exercise in which the patient shortens or contracts large muscle groups, thereby causing an increase in cardiac output, rather than by isometric or static exercise in which the muscle groups are tensed but not shortened, leading to disproportional increases in the patient's blood pressure that may impose a dangerous load on the left ventricle [19]. Most modern stress test laboratories employ either a bicycle or treadmill ergometer.

As the patient exercises, heart rate, blood pressure, and contractile state of the myocardium increase causing an increase in myocardial oxygen consumption [31]. To meet this increased metabolic demand, coronary blood flow increases proportionally—in normal persons by vasodilation of the coronary arterioles and capillaries where the main resistance to coronary blood flow occurs [18]. The extent of vasodilation depends upon the accumulation of the by-products of muscle metabolism. In patients with fixed coronary obstruction, however, the distal coronary bed dilates, but the chief resistance to coronary blood flow is now shifted proximally and, being fixed, cannot respond to the metabolic load imposed by exercise. Thus at some point during the exercise test, the oxygen demand exceeds the oxygen supply, and the resulting myocardial ischemia becomes manifest by symptoms or signs such as chest pain or ST-segment depression. It is important to emphasize that exercise-induced ST-segment depression is a functional manifestation of an electrophysiologic abnormality usually indicating that myocardial oxygen demand has exceeded the ability of coronary arteries to supply the increased oxygen needs [5]. The presence of this electrocardiographic abnormality is not always due to the presence of coronary artery disease, as there are diseases such as aortic stenosis or hypertension which may cause excessive oxygen demand and, thus, ischemic ST-segment depression without the presence of fixed coronary stenoses.

Predictive Accuracy of Exercise Testing

The predictive value of a test is the likelihood that disease is present or absent depending upon whether the test is positive or negative, respectively. With reference to the electrocardiographic response to exercise testing, the following is the definition of predictive value:

$$\text{Predictive value } (\%) = \frac{TP}{TP + PN} \times 100 \qquad (2.1)$$

$$\text{or } \frac{TN}{TN + FN} \times 100$$

where:

FN (false negative) = negative exercise ECG and positive angiogram;

FP (false positive) = positive exercise ECG and negative angiogram;

TN (true negative) = negative exercise ECG and negative
                       angiogram;

TP (true positive) = positive exercise ECG and positive
                       angiogram.

The sensitivity and specificity determine how accurate certain test results will be (that is, the predictive value). For example, if a positive exercise result was defined as a 2 mm ST-segment depression, rather than a 1 mm depression, the probability is very high that all individuals with positive test results will have significant coronary artery disease [35].

Another major determinant of the predictive accuracy of a test result is the prevalence of disease in the population under study or the likelihood of having disease before the test is undertaken [33]. This concept is referred to as Bayes theorem or the statistical law of conditional probability which states that the likelihood of disease after a diagnostic test (the post-test risk) cannot be entirely estimated from the test results but also requires knowledge of the prevalence of disease (pretest risk) of the individual in question [8,23,24]. Thus the predictive accuracy of any test outcome that is less than a perfect diagnostic test (that is, less than 100% specific) is influenced by the pretest likelihood of disease and the criteria used to define a test result. This concept is illustrated in table 2-1. Using the same test outcome (with a sensitivity and specificity of 95%), the predictive value (that is, the post-test likelihood of disease) would be 99% in an individual where the estimated prevalence of disease is 90%, as in patients with classical angina pectoris. However, the identical test outcome in an individual whose estimated prevalence of disease is 2%, such as in those individuals who are asymptomatic, would only be 28%. The same concepts hold true for a negative test outcome [16].

**The Coronary Artery Surgery Study on
Symptomatic Individuals**

To test the hypothesis that the diagnostic accuracy of stress testing is influenced by the prevalence of coronary artery disease, a recently reported study in a large cohort of men and women undergoing coronary arteriography for the evaluation of chest pain was completed [36]. The patient population was derived from 15 participating centers broadly distributed throughout the United States and Canada and consisted of 1,465 men and 580 women. All patients underwent graded exercise testing using the Bruce protocol and cardiac catheterization. The exercise test was considered positive when there was at least 1 mm of ST-segment depression or elevation. Significant coronary artery disease was defined as at least 70% narrowing

Table 2-1

Dependency of the Predictive Value on the Prevalence of Coronary Disease in Two Populations (n = 1000 patients each) Using a Test Result of 95% Sensitivity and 95% Specificity

	Population with Prevalence of 90%			Population with Prevalence of 2%		
	Subjects	Number with Positive Test	Number with Negative Test	Subjects	Number with Positive Test	Number with Negative Test
With disease	900	855	45	20	19	1
Without disease	100	5	95	980	49	931
Total	1000	860	140	1000	68	932
Predictive value						
Positive test		$\dfrac{855}{860} = 99\%$			$\dfrac{19}{68} = 28\%$	
Negative test			$\dfrac{95}{140} = 68\%$			$\dfrac{931}{932} = 99\%$

of the diameter of at least one major coronary segment. All patients had chest pain complaints which were categorized into three groups: definite angina, probable angina, and nonischemic chest pain. Excluded from the analysis were individuals with unstable angina, with previous myocardial infarction, on digitalis therapy at the time of the test, and asymptomatic individuals and those who failed to reach 85% of the maximum predicted heart rate in conjunction with a negative exercise test.

The results of the study are summarized in table 2-2. This group of patients with bothersome chest pain, representative of the individuals a clinician would probably subject to stress testing for additional information, demonstrated a 67% prevalence of coronary artery disease in men and 28% in women. While the predictive value of a positive exercise test was 88% for men, who had a high prevalence of coronary artery disease, it was only 46% for women, as might be expected from their lower prevalence of coronary artery disease.

As can be seen from table 2-2, the predictive value of a positive exercise test decreased as the prevalence of coronary disease in the population under question decreased. Conversely, the predictive value of a negative exercise test increased as the prevalence of disease decreased. When individuals in whom the prevalence of coronary artery disease is high (for example, definite angina) were tested, a positive exercise test only slightly increased an already high prevalence of coronary artery disease; whereas a negative test was more likely to be falsely negative. On the other hand, when individuals in whom the prevalence of disease was low (for example, women with nonischemic pain) were tested, a negative exercise test only confirmed an already low likelihood of disease, and a positive exercise test was more likely to be falsely positive.

Thus, before the results of exercise testing can be objectively evaluated, the pretest risk of coronary disease (or the prevalence of coronary disease) must first be considered. The preceding study only dealt with symptomatic patients coming to the exercise laboratory for the diagnosis of coronary artery disease.

Previous Studies in Asymptomatic Individuals

Asymptomatic individuals would be expected to have a low probability of disease before the results of exercise testing. The predictive value of a positive electrocardiographic response to exercise would also be expected to be quite low. In the three studies cited in table 2-3, the predictive value of a positive electrocardiographic response to exercise ranged from 25% to 64% [3,11,12].

Table 2-2
Pretest Risk of Coronary Disease and Predictive Value of a Positive and Negative Exercise Test in the Coronary Artery Surgery Study

History	Sex	Number	Pretest Risk of Coronary Disease (%)	Predictive Value (%)	
				+ET[a]	−ET[b]
Definite angina	Male	620	89	96	35
Definite angina	Female	98	62	73	67
Probable angina	Male	594	70	87	56
Probable angina	Female	240	40	54	78
Nonischemic pain	Male	251	22	39	86
Nonischemic pain	Female	242	5	6	95

[a]Predictive value of a positive exercise test (+ET) = percentage of positive results that are truly positive.
[b]Predictive value of a negative test (−ET) = percentage of negative results that are truly negative.

Table 2–3
Predictive Value of a Positive Electrocardiographic Response to Exercise in Asymptomatic Individuals

Study	Predictive Value (%)
Borer et al. [3]	37
Froelicher et al. [12]	25
Erikssen et al. [11]	64

Conclusions

Before using the exercise test as a screening procedure for coronary artery disease, one should recognize that its diagnostic accuracy is very limited. In an asymptomatic individual, a positive electrocardiographic response to exercise is much more likely to be found than in an individual with normal coronary arteries, and even a negative exercise response does not rule out severe coronary disease.

This recent recognition of the diagnostic limitations of electrocardiographic exercise testing has led other investigators to study different exercise test variables to increase the predictive accuracy of the exercise test [17,35]. These variables include amount [14,27], onset and duration of ST-segment depression [15], the duration of exercise [21], the number of leads causing ST-segment depression [6], exertional hypotension [22,32], poor heart-rate response to exercise [9], exercise-induced chest pain [34], and the R-wave response to exercise [2]. Although these additional variables have been shown to be of great value in symptomatic patients, none has been tested in asymptomatic individuals in whom the prevalence of coronary artery disease is low. Moreover, the increased predictive accuracy of the exercise test might still occur at the expense of a decreased sensitivity [35] so that fewer patients with coronary artery disease would be detected using these newer exercise variables. Perhaps the best way to increase the diagnostic accuracy of exercise testing is to consider it to be an extension of the clinical and risk-factor evaluation of a patient and to use ST-segment changes not to provide a yes-or-no statement regarding the presence of coronary artery disease but to yield a probability statement based on a continuum of risk [8,10,24,28]. If the asymptomatic individual has an intermediate risk of coronary disease after an exercise electrocardiographic test result, another independent noninvasive test such as an exercise thallium test [25], a radionuclide cineangiography [4], or a cardiokymography [29] can be utilized to further increase or reduce the risk of coronary artery disease.

Finally, the exercise test might be used to yield other important information prior to an exercise program. The exercise capacity could be quantitated and repeated after an exercise program to document improvement. If exercise-induced ST-segment depression or arrhythmias occur, the patient could be shown how to take his pulse rate during exercise and prevent it from exceeding the heart rate which caused the abnormalities during the exercise test. In this way, the physician can be provided with a more rational basis from which to advise about exercise.

References

1. Bartel, A.G., Behar, V.S., Peter, R.H., Orgain, E.S., and Kong, Y. Graded exercise stress test in angiographically documented coronary artery diseases. *Circulation* 49:348–356, 1974.

2. Bonoris, P.E., Greenberg, P.S., Castellanet, M.J., and Ellestad, M.H. Significance of changes in R-wave amplitude during treadmill stress testing: Angiographic correlation. *Am. J. Cardiol.* 41:846–851, 1978.

3. Borer, J.S., Brensike, J.F., Redwood, D.R., et al. Limitations of the electrocardiographic response to exercise in predicting coronary-artery disease. *N. Engl. J. Med.* 293:367–371, 1975.

4. Borer, J.S., Kent, K.M., Bacharach, S.L., et al. Sensitivity, specificity, and predictive accuracy of radionuclide cineangiography during exercise in patients with coronary artery disease: Comparison with exercise electrocardiography. *Circulation* 60:572–590, 1979.

5. Bruce, R.A. Values and limitations of exercise electrocardiography. *Circulation* 50:1–3, 1974.

6. Chaitman, B.R., Waters, D.D., Bourassa, M.G., Tubau, J.F., Wagniart, P., and Ferguson, R.J. The importance of clinical subsets in interpreting maximal treadmill exercise test results: The role of multiple-lead ECG systems. *Circulation* 59:560–570, 1979.

7. Detry, J.M.R., Kapita, B.M., Cosyns, J., Sottiaux, B., Brasseur, L.A., and Rousseau, M.F. Diagnostic value of history and maximal exercise electrocardiography in men and women suspected of coronary heart disease. *Circulation* 56:756–761, 1977.

8. Diamond, G.A., and Forrester, J.S., Analysis of probability as an aid in the clinical diagnosis of coronary disease. *N. Engl. J. Med.* 300:1350–1358, 1979.

9. Ellestad, M.H., and Wan, M.K.C. Predictive implications of stress testing. *Circulation* 51:363–369, 1975.

10. Epstein, S.E. Implications of probability analysis on the strategy used for noninvasive detection of coronary disease. *Am. J. Cardiol.* 46:491–499, 1980.

11. Erikssen, J., Enge, I., Forfang, K., and Storstein, O. False positive diagnostic tests and coronary angiographic findings in 105 presumably healthy males. *Circulation* 54:371–376, 1976.

12. Froelicher, V.F., Jr., Thompson, A.J., Longo, M.R., Jr., Triebwasser, J.H., and Lancaster, M.C. Value of exercise testing for screening asymptomatic men in latent coronary disease. *Prog. Cardiov. Dis.* 18:265–276, 1976.

13. Froelicher, V.F., Jr., Yanowitz, F.G., Thompson, A.J., and Lancaster, M.C. The correlation of coronary angiography and the electro-cardiographic response to maximal treadmill testing in 76 asymptomatic men. *Circulation* 48:597–604, 1973.

14. Goldman, S., Tselos, S., and Cohn, K. Marked depth of ST-segment depression during treadmill exercise testing: Indicator of severe coronary artery disease. *Chest* 69:729–733, 1976.

15. Goldschlager, N., Selzer, A., and Cohn, K. Treadmill stress tests as indicators of presence and severity of coronary artery disease. *Ann. Intern. Med.* 85:277–286, 1976.

16. Gorry, G.A., Pauker, S.G., and Swartz, W.B. The diagnostic importance of the normal finding. *N. Engl. J. Med.* 298:486–489, 1978.

17. Hollenberg, M., Budge, W.R., Wisneski, J.A., and Gertz, E.W. Treadmill score quantifies electrocardiographic response to exercise and improves test accuracy and reproducibility. *Circulation* 61:276–285, 1980.

18. Kitamura, K., Jorgensen, C.R., Gobel, F.L., Taylor, H.L., and Wang, Y. Hemodynamic correlates of myocardial oxygen consumption during upright exercise. *J. Appl. Physiol.* 32:516–522, 1972.

19. Mathews, O.A., Atkins, J.M., Houston, J.D., Blomqvist, G., and Mullins, C.B. Arrhythmias induced by isometric exercise (handgrip). *Clin. Res.* 19:23, 1971.

20. McConahay, D.R., McCallister, B.D., and Smith, R.E. Post-exercise electrocardiography: Correlations with coronary arteriography and left ventricular hemodynamics. *Am. J. Cardiol.* 28:1–9, 1971.

21. McNeer, J.E., Margolis, J.R., Lee, K.L., et al. The role of the exercise test in the evaluation of patients for ischemic heart disease. *Circulation* 57:64–70, 1978.

22. Morris, S.M., Phillips, J.F., Jordan, J.W., and McHenry, P.L. Incidence and significance of decreases in systolic blood pressure during graded exercise testing. *Am. J. Cardiol.* 41:221–226, 1977.

23. Redwood, D.R., Borer, J.S., and Epstein, S.E. Whither the ST-segment during exercise? *Circulation* 54:703–706, 1976.

24. Rifkin, R.D., and Hood, W.B., Jr. Bayesian analysis of electrocardiographic stress testing. *N. Engl. J. Med.* 297:681–686, 1977.

25. Ritchie, J.L., Zaret, B.L., Strauss, H.W., et al. Myocardial imaging with thallium-201: A multicenter study in patients with angina pectoris or acute myocardial infarction. *Am. J. Cardiol.* 42:345–350, 1978.

26. Roitman, D., Jones, W.B., and Sheffield, L.T. Comparison of submaximal exercise ECG test with coronary cineangiocardiogram. *Ann. Intern. Med.* 72:641–647, 1970.

27. Sanmarco, M.E., Pontius, S., and Selvester, R.H. Abnormal blood pressure response and marked ischemic ST-segment depression as predictors of severe coronary disease. *Circulation* 61:572–578, 1980.

28. Selzer, A., Cohn, K., and Goldschlager, N. On the interpretation of the exercise test. *Circulation* 58:193–195, 1978.

29. Silverberg, R.A., Diamond, G.A., Vas, R., Tzivoni, D., Swan, H.J.C., Forrester, J.S. Noninvasive diagnosis of coronary artery disease: The cardiokymographic stress test. *Circulation* 61:579–589, 1980.

30. Sketch, M.H., Mohiuddin, S.M., Lynch, J.D., Zencka, A.E., and Runco, V. Significant sex differences in the correlation of electrocardiographic exercise testing and coronary arteriograms. *Am. J. Cardiol.* 36:169–173, 1975.

31. Sonnenblick, E.H., Ross, J., Jr., and Braunwald, E. Oxygen consumption of the heart: Newer concepts of its multifactorial determination. *Am. J. Cardiol.* 22:328–336, 1968.

32. Thomson, P.D., and Keelman, M.H. Hypotension accompanying the onset of exertional angina. *Circulation* 52:28–32, 1975.

33. Vecchio, T.J. Predictive value of a single diagnostic test in unselected populations. *N. Engl. J. Med.* 274:1171–1173, 1966.

34. Weiner, D.A., McCabe, C.H., Hueter, D.C., Ryan, J.T., and Hood, W.B., Jr. The predictive value of anginal chest pain as an indicator of coronary disease during exercise testing. *Am. Heart. J.* 96:458–462, 1978.

35. Weiner, D.A., McCabe, C.H., Ryan, T.J. Identification of patients with left main and three vessel coronary disease with clinical and exercise test variables. *Am. J. Cardiol.* 46:21–27, 1980.

36. Weiner, D.A., Ryan, T.J., McCabe, C.H., et al. Exercise stress testing: Correlations among history of angina, ST-segment response and prevalence of coronary-artery disease in the Coronary Artery Surgery Study (CASS). *N. Engl. J. Med.* 301:230–235, 1979.

3 Compliance and Addiction to Exercise

Michael L. Sachs, Ph.D.

The concept of the exercising adult assumes a person who is participating in physical activity. Any number of motivational factors may underlie this participation. Additionally, the particular instance of exercising in which we view a given individual may be one occasion in a regular, systematic program of physical activity, or it may be a relatively isolated occurrence.

Although polls have indicated that millions of people participate in physical activity [17], with a fair percentage of these participating on a regular basis, there is still considerable room for improvement in the percentage of people who engage *regularly* in vigorous exercise. The critical concern for those individuals who only participate irregularly, or who are just starting an exercise program, is compliance or adherence to the activity. The motivational factors required to stimulate people to begin a program of exercise are a separate topic of consideration. Once a person has initiated a program of exercise, it is the sports medicine professional's goal to structure programs for that individual which facilitate adherence to the activity.

Adherence involves sticking with exercise. The issue of compliance has been dealt with extensively in the medical literature [8,11]. The body of literature on adherence to physical activity, although less voluminous, has been increasing recently in both quantity and quality. Of particular interest are works by Dishman and his colleagues [7] as well as other sources [4,16,18,21,22].

——The dropout rate in exercise programs ranges widely, from 1.2% to 95%, with most dropout rates ranging from 30% to 70% of the participants in the programs [18]. These figures, however, provide no indication of the percentages for individuals who begin (and perhaps end) exercising on their own without the benefits (or drawbacks) of an organized exercise program.

Dishman cites a number of factors that have been suggested as significant in adherence to exercise: attitudes toward physical activity, self-perceptions of exercise ability, and feelings of health responsibility. These factors have been shown, however, not to be significant in predicting adherence although they may be important in determining initial involvement in physical activity [5–7].

A number of additional factors have been shown to be associated with adherence. Remaining free of injuries is of particular importance. Continued participation is impossible if injuries hinder or eliminate the opportunity to engage in physical activity. A second factor of note is the role of significant others. Participants whose spouses had favorable attitudes toward the program had considerably better patterns of adherence than participants whose spouses had neutral or negative attitudes [12].

The location of the exercise facility represents a third factor. In one study, participants had campus offices significantly closer to the testing/ exercise facilities than nonparticipants [10]. Teraslinna et al. [31] found, similarly, that those willing to participate in an exercise program lived nearer to the exercise facility than those unwilling to participate. Certainly, if convenience is important to the individual, making it easier to engage in physical activity should increase the possibility of continuing participation.

The attainment of exercise objectives is of particular importance. Danielson and Wanzel found that those individuals who did not attain their objectives tended to drop out of the exercise program much faster than those who did obtain their objectives [4]. Setting reasonable, attainable goals in any situation usually leads to increased satisfaction with that situation, enhancing the likelihood of continued participation.

Additionally, the health status of participants has been shown to be related to adherence. Patients with a disability associated with disease, such as cardiovascular problems, are more inclined to adhere to a treatment program.

Dishman has pointed out that while factors such as those cited may be associated with adherence to exercise, they have not been shown to be useful in predicting adherence [5]. Since a major goal is to be able to predict who will adhere and who will drop out, this concern takes on added importance.

Accordingly, Dishman et al. attempted to develop a psychobiologic model in diagnosing dropout proneness [7]. They found three factors—self-motivation, percent body fat, and body weight—that were significant in predicting dropout proneness. Knowledge of these three variables "permitted accurate classification of participants into actual adherence or dropout groups for approximately 80% of the cases." Furthermore, employing these three variables in the regression equation provided a multiple correlation of 0.67, which accounts for a considerable portion ($R^2 = 0.45$) of the variance in adherence behavior.

It might, therefore, be said that individuals who are heavy, have a high percentage of body fat, and lack self-motivation have a high probability of quitting. One might note, particularly, the clinical and practical significance of these factors. They are all easily and reliably assessed. Self-motivation inventory has been constructed by Dishman et al. [7]. One might recommend, therefore, that exercise programs consider using this model in evaluating participants in their programs, perhaps attempting to improve on or modify the model to meet their particular needs.

Dishman has identified other areas of importance in considering adherence to exercise [5–7]. Situational characteristics are significant in facilitating adherence. The presence or absence of social reinforcements that may be derived from interpersonal relationships that develop between exercisers or with an exercise leader or other program staff are potentially significant in adherence. This consideration relates to the earlier findings of Heinzelmann and Bagley [12], as well as Jones and Jones [14], concerning the importance of reinforcements from significant others in the person's environment. In addition to these significant others, those individuals in the exercise situation can play an important role in facilitating adherence.

Where possible, personal exercise prescription based on behavioral tailoring will provide a program ideally suited to a given individual's needs. In particular, this may help achieve the development and attainment of reasonable exercise objectives. Self-monitoring of exercise behavior, such as daily record keeping, is an effective technique in behavioral management that may provide frequent reinforcement to the individual.

In addition to tailoring the program to meet the needs of the individual, the exercise setting can sometimes be modified to accommodate the exerciser; frequently both the setting and the exerciser need to be modified. For example, running on a track may prove difficult for some (because it is particularly boring), so working with the individual to divide time between the track and trails through neighboring areas (particularly woods) may enhance the possibility of adherence. Certainly, there are many cognitive-behavioral strategies, such as self-statements, cognitive rehearsal, self-efficacy, attribution, shaping, and stimulus control that may facilitate maintenance of exercise behavior [2].

Exercise behavior should become directly or concretely reinforcing for the individual—otherwise, the behavior will be extinguished rapidly, and another dropout will be added to the statistics. One reinforcement of particular note is the famous feel-better phenomenon, which Morgan found to be reported by 85% of exercise participants while exercising [18]. Although not always demonstrable on psychologic or physiologic tests, this almost universal phenomenon is one that should be highlighted and enhanced where possible.

One can cite, therefore, a number of general strategies for facilitating adherence: use of group settings, the convenient accessibility of exercise settings, the support of significant others, limitation of the intensity of the exercise so that it is not stressful to the point of injury, and the attainment of training objectives. These strategies will be employed in the most thorough programs. In addition, three other steps may be used to facilitate exercise adherence. First, initial diagnosis of the dropout-prone individual, perhaps using the model of Dishman et al. will be of value [7]. Attempts to tie in personality profiles of dropouts may prove of interest to some program leaders. Second, subsequent determination of influences within the exercise setting to which the individual might be sensitive will enhance the use of strategies in modifying the setting to highlight these critical influences. Finally, the appropriate manipulation of these situational factors to enhance the likelihood of adherence will provide the highest probability of having an exercise program with a high rate of adherence of the participants.

Within the context of considering adherence to exercise, the subject of exercise addiction becomes important. Addiction to exercise, and to running in particular, has received considerable attention since William Glasser's book on *Positive Addiction* [9].

It might be appropriate to note, however, that the term addiction is not the preferred one. Indeed, in 1964 the World Health Organization, noting the abuse of the terms drug addiction and drug habituation, suggested replacement of these terms with the term drug dependence [33]. The term addiction has so many different popular uses that it is often difficult to clarify exactly what is meant by the word. Moreover, use of the term addiction with respect to exercise has received criticism from some authorities who suggest that associating these two concepts is inappropriate [3]. However, the term addiction has remained in popular usage, and while it might be preferable to use a term such as dependence upon exercise, the term addiction will be used herein.

Addiction is a process, rather than a condition. Peele has noted that addiction is not characteristic of drugs or activities per se but of the involvement that a person forms with these substances or events [23]. A person can indeed become addicted to exercise, just as individuals can become addicted to drugs, smoking, meditation, or television.

Glasser's work popularized the concept that addictions can be good for the individual and can provide strength, as opposed to weakening the person. Glasser examined activities such as running and meditation which are supportive of the individual's psychology and physiology. These positive addictions are suggested as providing psychologic strength and increasing the satisfaction derived from life. The thesis of Glasser's work is that "many people, weak and strong, can help themselves to be stronger, and an important new path to strength may be positive addiction" [9].

Descriptions of the positive addiction state provided by Glasser include a loss of the sense of oneself, floating, euphoria, and a total integration with running. Indeed, the positive addiction state identified by Glasser is closely related to experiences known as the runner's high. Glasser recommends running for any individual, psychologically strong or weak, who desires a positively addicting activity [9].

Research evidence on exercise addiction, however, is limited because of the relative newness of the concept and the difficulty of studying addicted exercisers, particularly in an experimental context. Baekeland, for example, could not get regular exercisers to stop exercising for any amount of money [1]. It is virtually impossible to get addicted exercisers to stop for any significant length of time (more than a day or two), which would be needed to provide information that could be evaluated critically. When addicted runners are forced to stop, which occurs when they are injured, the compounding effect of this injury, or other factors, poses significant difficulties for any findings about addiction to the activity.

Sachs and Pargman provided a definition of addiction to exercise: "addiction, of a psychological and/or physiological nature, upon a regular regimen of physical activity, characterized by withdrawal symptoms after 24–36 hours without exercise" [29]. The exact amount of time depends on the individual. The withdrawal symptoms are critical in the determination of the presence or absence and degree of addiction to exercise. These symptoms will become evident in addicted individuals if they do not or cannot exercise on a day when they had originally planned to do so. For example, a runner who regularly takes days off on Sundays and Wednesdays does not expect to run on those days and would not be expected to develop withdrawal symptoms at those times. However, if this individual had expected to run on a Saturday, and for some reason was unable to do so, then one would expect withdrawal symptoms to develop.

These withdrawal symptoms include anxiety, restlessness, guilt, irritability, tension, bloatedness, muscle twitching, and discomfort. Although these symptoms are primarily psychologic in nature, a number of physiologic reactions have been noted. Sachs, however, found that the degree of symptomatology reported by a group of runners was only low to moderate [28]. Joseph has noted that women are more likely to associate themselves with withdrawal symptoms than men, perhaps due to supposedly greater sensitivity or willingness to report symptoms [15]. Although anecdotal reports suggest high levels of such symptoms as guilt or anxiety in the individual deprived of exercise, it is possible that such symptoms will not be reported with a similar level of intensity on paper and pencil tests.

Exercisers, such as runners, have reported developing addiction to their activity in as little as one to two months [28], although Glasser suggests that up to two years may be required [9]. Sachs noted that some of the runners in his study reported periods of 5, 10, and even 20 years before addiction to the activity was felt to be present [25].

Although numerous studies have dealt with motivation for beginning participation and note such factors as influences from other individuals, concerns of general health, improvement of cardiovascular fitness, and body weight reduction, the process by which addiction develops has not yet been identified in runners. Neither Sachs [25], Sachs and Pargman [29], nor Jacobs [13], in three separate studies which attempted to identify this process, uncovered a personality typology of runners or a general descriptive categorization of the addictive process.

Addiction to exercise, and to running in particular, is not always positive in nature. Morgan has identified the negatively addicting aspects of exercise [19,20]. Morgan cites a number of case studies of runners who are virtually consumed by the need to run and alter their daily schedules dramatically, continue to run when seriously injured, and neglect the responsibilities of work, home, and family. Symptoms of negative addiction cited include decreased ability to concentrate, lapses in judgment, listlessness, fatigue, constant thought about running, impaired social and work activity, and skipping appointments because of the need to run.

In the negatively addicted participant, exercise has moved from an important but considered aspect of the person's existence to a controlling factor, eliminating other choices in life. The concept of control is critical because the positively addicted runner has control over the activity while the negative addict has progressed to the point where the activity controls the person.

Whether dependence on exercise is truly an addiction or is nothing more than a glorified habit, the general concept is of particular importance to those sports medicine professionals concerned with adherence to physical activity. Further work in examining addiction to exercise will identify those factors significant in the process of the development of addiction and may help identify those individuals most likely to become addicted. Both of these areas are important because the professional can use the information available to establish an addictive relationship of the individual with the activity of exercise. According to Peele's concept, addiction is characteristic of the involvement a person forms with particular substances or events [23]. The professional who can facilitate this involvement has virtually assured that the individual will adhere to the activity.

Although continued involvement with an activity may, for a small percentage of addicted exercisers, lead to negative addiction, the level of addiction for the vast majority of participants will be a positive one. In Glasser's terms, involvement in the activity will provide both psychologic and physiologic strength for the person [9]. Certainly, the initial stages that the professional is concerned with are the beginning levels of positive addiction to the activity.

By familiarizing oneself with the literature available on addiction to exercise as well as delving in related areas of importance, such as the runner's high, the sports medicine professional will be prepared with information providing a greater understanding of these concepts and their potential significance in the drive to increase adherence to physical activity.

References

1. Baekeland, F. Exercise deprivation: Sleep and psychological reactions. *Arch. Gen. Psychiatry* 22:365–369, 1970.

2. Buffone, G.W., Sachs, M.L., and Dowd, E.T. Cognitive-behavioral strategies for facilitating maintenance of exercise behavior. In M.H. Sacks and M.L. Sachs (Eds.), *Running Therapy.* Champaign, Ill.: Human Kinetics Publishers. In press.

3. Cooper, A. Running and narcissism. Presented at the Third Annual Psychology of Running Seminar. Cornell University Medical College, New York, October 24, 1980.

4. Danielson, R.R., and Wanzel, R.S. Exercise objectives of fitness program dropouts. In D.M. Landers and R.W. Christina (Eds.), *Psychology of Motor Behavior and Sport, 1977.* Champaign, Ill.: Human Kinetics Publishers, 1978.

5. Dishman, R.K. Biologic influences on exercise adherence. *J. Cardiac Rehabilitation.* In press.

6. Dishman, R.K. Prediction of adherence to habitual physical activity. In H.J. Montoye and F.J. Nagle (Eds.), *Exercise in Health and Disease.* Springfield, Ill.: Charles C. Thomas, 1981.

7. Dishman, R.K., Ickes, W.J., and Morgan, W.P. Self-motivation and adherence to habitual physical activity. *J. Appl. Social Psychology* 10:115–131, 1980.

8. Dunbar, J.M., and Stunkard, J.A. Adherence to diet and drug regimen. In R. Levy, B. Rifkind, B. Dennis, and N. Ernst (Eds.), *Nutrition, Lipids, and Coronary Heart Disease.* New York: Raven Press, 1979.

9. Glasser, William. *Positive Addiction.* New York: Harper and Row, 1976.

10. Hanson, M.G. Coronary heart disease, exercise, and motivation in middle-aged males. Ph.D. dissertation, University of Wisconsin, 1976.

11. Haynes, R.B., Taylor, D.W., and Sackett, D.L. *Compliance in Health Care.* Baltimore: Johns Hopkins University Press, 1979.

12. Heinzelmann, F., and Bagley, R.W. Response to physical activity programs and their effects on health behavior. *Public Health Rep.* 85:905–911, 1970.

13. Jacobs, L.W. Running as an addiction process. Ph.D. dissertation, University of Alberta, 1980.

14. Jones, S.B., and Jones, D.C. Serious jogging and family life: Marathon and sub-marathon running. Presented at the annual meeting of the American Sociological Association. Chicago, Ill., September 5–9, 1977.

15. Joseph, P. The running commitment and work satisfaction. Presented at the Third Annual Psychology of Running Seminar. Cornell University Medical College, New York, October 24, 1980.

16. Massie, J., and Shephard, R. Physiological and psychological effects of training. *Med. Sci. Sports* 3:110–117, 1971.

17. Moore, K. Taking part: You ain't seen nothin' yet. *Sports Illustrated* 49, no. 26:38–48, December 25, 1978 to January 1, 1979.

18. Morgan, W.P. Involvement in vigorous physical activity with special reference to adherence. *Proceedings of the NCPEAM/NAPECW National Conference,* 1977. Pp. 235–246.

19. Morgan, W.P. Negative addiction in runners. *Phys. Sports Med.* 7, no. 2:56–63, 67–70, February 1979.

20. Morgan, W.P. Running into addiction. *The Runner* 1, no. 6:72–74, 76, March 1979.

21. Oldridge, N.B. Compliance in exercise rehabilitation. *Phys. Sports Med.* 7:94–103, 1979.

22. Oldridge, N.B., Wicks, J.R., Hanley, V.C., Sutton, J.R., and Jones, N.L. Noncompliance in an exercise rehabilitation program for men who have suffered a myocardial infarction. *Can. Med. Assoc. J.* 118:361–364, 1978.

23. Peele, S. Addiction: The analgesic experience. *Human Nature* 1, no. 9:61–67, September 1978.

24. Pollock, M.O., Gettman, L.R., Milesis, C.A., et al. Effects of frequency and duration of training on attrition and incidence of injury. *Med. Sci. Sports* 9:31–36, 1977.

25. Sachs, M.L. An examination of the relationship of commitment to and dependence upon running to a model for participation in running and personality typology of regular runners. Unpublished manuscript, Florida State University, 1979.

26. Sachs, M.L. On the trail of the runner's high: A descriptive and experimental investigation of characteristics of an elusive phenomenon. Ph.D. dissertation, Florida State University, 1980.

27. Sachs, M.L. The runner's high. Presented at the Third Annual Psychology of Running Seminar. Cornell University Medical College, New York, October 24, 1980.

28. Sachs, M.L. Running addiction. In M.H. Sacks and M.L. Sachs (Eds.), *Running Therapy.* Champaign, Ill.: Human Kinetics Publishers. In press.

29. Sachs, M.L., and Pargman, D. Running addiction: A depth interview examination. *J. Sport Behavior* 2, no. 3:143–155, 1979.

30. Sacks, M.H. Running addiction. Presented at the Third Annual Psychology of Running Seminar. Cornell University Medical College, New York, October 24, 1980.

31. Teraslinna, P., Partanen, T., Oja, P., and Koskela, A. Some social characteristics and living habits associated with willingness to participate in a physical activity intervention study. *J. Sports Med. Phys. Fitness* 10:138–144, 1970.

32. Thirer, J. Distinguishing the successful runner from the running drop-out. Presented at the Third Annual Psychology of Running Seminar. Cornell University Medical College, New York, October 24, 1980.

33. Worick, W.W., and Schaller, W.E. *Alcohol, Tobacco and Drugs: Their Use and Abuse.* Englewood Cliffs, N.J.: Prentice-Hall, 1977.

Fitness Centers

4

Corporate Fitness Centers

Richard G. Day
with the assistance of
Robert C. Cantu, M.D.

The concept of corporate fitness had its origins at the Institute for Working Physiology in Stockholm, Sweden in the nineteenth century. The motivating force was not the health of workers, but how much work could be extracted from them. Forty-five percent of maximal oxygen consumption was determined to be the maximal effort an individual could sustain for eight hours, return home functional, and be able to rise the next day for a similar work effort. Precise maximal work loads for various jobs could thus be prescribed.

Industry in the United States is reintroducing work physiology to the employee in the form of cardiovascular exercise programs. The ever-growing list of private firms committed to employee fitness includes Arco, Boeing, Bonnie Bell, Bose, Chase Manhattan, Exxon, Firestone, Ford Motor Company, General Foods, Goodyear, Kimberly-Clark, Merrill Lynch, Metropolitan Life, Norton Company, Pepsico, Phillips Petroleum, Polaroid, Rockwell International, Sentry Insurance, Sly, Spaulding, Western Electric, and Xerox. The incentive to industry is reduced illness and absenteeism, less employee turnover, and greater productivity.

The federal government is attempting to curtail ever upwardly spiraling health-care expenditures by promoting fitness and preventive medicine and heeding the words of the late John Knowles: "The next big advance in modern medicine will be in what the patient can do for himself." The Public Health Service's "Forward Plan" for 1977 to 1981 states, "Habitual inactivity is thought to contribute to hypertension, chronic fatigue, and resulting physical inefficiency, premature aging, poor musculature, and lack of flexibility which are the major causes of lower back pain and injury, mental tension, coronary heart disease, and obesity" [7].

Hospitals have become increasingly involved in the fitness movement. As Walter J. McNerney states, "A new direction is needed for our medical system...that should concentrate on positive health rather than simply curative treatment...more doctors and hospitals don't necessarily add up to better health. We are discovering that better health depends less on medicine than on life style, environment, and cultural factors" [5]. The good life can kill you was the finding of a recent report from the Massachusetts General Hospital which showed that three out of five hospitalizations could be avoided if people took better care of themselves [4]. The message is quite clear that an ounce of prevention is still worth a pound of cure, and far less expensive.

The exercising adult is no longer a strange animal. Only a very few years ago, however, if one was seen running in the streets, that person was likely to receive many catcalls and less than pleasant gestures from irritated passersby or motorists. Why were these people running, bicycling, and walking? The answer can be found in physical education, but most of these programs focused their attention on the healthy elite. The majority of people are represented by the physically disadvantaged. The physically disadvantaged are those people who need special care and consideration while exercising. Included in this group are those with cardiovascular, respiratory, diabetic, overweight, orthopedic, visual, auditory, motor, sensory, or mental deficiencies, plus the aged [2].

Employee Health Enhancement at Sentry Insurance

There are many programs within hospitals, universities, and even corporations which provide a structured, safe program, allowing everyone to enjoy the benefits of exercise. At Sentry Insurance, the program is designed for a holistic approach to help the employees achieve a higher level of wellness. The Sentry Employee Health Enhancement Program began in 1977 and is more than a physical fitness facility. The chief executive officer, John Joanis, realized the importance of employee health when he experienced the benefits of a weight loss and exercise program himself.

The goal of the program is to keep employees healthy so their ability to work efficiently is not hindered by an illness-related problem. In theory, if a person is healthy and misses fewer days of work, job productivity will increase. The thought is not to milk the employee to work harder and faster but rather to reduce human error and increase efficiency. Ultimately, there should also be a decrease in health claims as employees attain a higher level of wellness. This should lead to lower employee-insurance premiums, an incentive itself.

A major problem today is the rapidly increasing cost of health care. From 1965 to 1978, the National Health Expenditure increased 340%, and the trend continues [3]. The per capita expenditure in 1978 was $735 [9]. What will it be by 1990? It appears that it is out of control and something must be done. People must take responsibility for their health, and incentives must be provided so they will.

Sentry is committed to helping the employee achieve higher levels of wellness. The program goes beyond helping just the active participants as benefits are provided that reach all employees. Sentry's environment supports and encourages people to become well through no-smoking areas, the monthly health newsletter (*Fit Lines*), plus access to both the fitness facility as well as a quiet room. The quiet room has soft furniture and subtle lighting to enhance employee relaxation. It is not meant for work breaks. If employees feel a need to go to the quiet room, they just tell their supervisor and stay for as long as needed, usually 5 to 15 minutes.

The program provides T-shirts, certificates, verbal encouragement, and other awards as incentives to participate. Every employee, not just executives or management, is encouraged to participate in the programs. In order to effectively modify the lifestyle of employees, the significant others [8] are also encouraged to participate. This provides a support group so that all will be working toward a common goal. The significant others include spouse, children, or a friend if one is single. Other conveniences include lockers, showers, towels, gym suits, sweat suits, hair dryers, and recreational equipment. In fact, the participant need only bring footwear.

Before employees may participate in a structured program, they must have medical clearance [1,6]. If they wish to use facilities on their own, that is, basketball, racquetball, and so forth, medical clearance, though encouraged, is not mandatory.

Since 1977 Sentry has established three centers: Sentry World Headquarters in Stevens Point, Wisconsin (1977); Sentry Center West in Scottsdale, Arizona (1977); and Sentry Center East in Concord, Massachusetts (1979). The programs vary in each of the Sentry facilities (see table 4-1). The geographic locations also have inherent difficulties unique to each program. Two of the Sentry complexes, Sentry World Headquarters and Sentry Center West, have the most elaborate facilities including racquetball courts, swimming pools, and a fitness laboratory with nautilus equipment. The exercise facilities at each location are listed in table 4-2. Because the facilities differ in size, staffing also differs, as seen in table 4-3, and programs vary (table 4-4).

To cope with the differences at Sentry Center East a unique arrangement was made with Emerson Hospital, which is directly across the street. An agreement was made through the efforts of Robert C. Cantu, M.D., director of the Service of Sports Medicine; Bernice McPhee, director of education and training at Emerson; Lucille Gervalini, R.N., the employee health nurse at Emerson; and Ronald J. Cook, Ph.D., national manager of Sentry Employee Health Enhancement. The idea was to combine existing programs at each institution in a complementary manner to maximize utilization with virtually no increase in cost to either party. Sentry provides the exercise facility and cardiovascular programs; Emerson provides the cardiopulmonary testing services, medical clearance, and employee-health lecture series. The following is a sample of what the health lecture series might include:

Stress	Diet and weight control
Common eye disorders	Cardiovascular health program
Loss and grief	Preparing for the holidays (alcohol)
Allergies and allergic reactions	
Fitness and exercise	Choosing and using a physician
How to insure a healthy, beautiful smile	Mid-life crisis
	Aging

Table 4–1
Employee Services at Sentry Centers

Employee Services	Sentry World Headquarters	Sentry Center West	Sentry Center East
Assertiveness training	•	•	•
Career counseling	•	•	•
Employee assistance	•	•	•
Environmental change (vacation)	•	•	•
Exercise program	•	•	•
Financial planning	•	•	•
Fit Lines (health newsletter)	•	•	•
Flex-time	•	•	•
Free expression of emotions	•	•	•
Issue awareness			•
Medical evaluation	•		
Nutrition	•	•	•
Protected parking area	•		
Quarterly information meetings	•	•	•
Quiet room	•	•	•
Rest	•	•	•
Spiritual activities and nourishment	•		

•Available at this site.

Table 4–2
Exercise Facilities at Sentry Centers

	Sentry World Headquarters	Sentry Center West	Sentry Center East
Gymnasium			
Badminton courts	•		•
Basketball courts	•	•	•
Tennis court			•
Volleyball court	•	•	•
Jogging	•	•	•
Fitness laboratory			
Treadmills	•	•	
Bicycle ergometers	•	•	•
Rowing machines	•	•	•
Jump ropes	•	•	•
Stretch area	•	•	•
Low beam	•	•	•
Nautilus equipment (full array)	•	•	
Swimming pool	•	•	
Racquetball courts	•	•	
Tennis courts (outdoor)		•	
Softball field		•	
Outdoor jogging routes	•	•	•

•Available at this site.

Table 4–3
Staffing at Sentry Centers

Center	Staff
Sentry World Headquarters	6 full-time 2 student interns 9 part-time
Sentry Center West	3 full-time 2 part-time
Sentry Center East	1 full-time

Table 4–4
Programming at Sentry Centers

	Sentry World Headquarters	Sentry Center West	Sentry Center East
Aerobic swimming	•	•	
Cardiovascular conditioning	•	•	•
Diet and exercise	•	•	•
Dance aerobics	•	•	•
General body conditioning	•	•	•
Low back program	•	•	
Blood pressure screening	•	•	•
Cardiovascular resuscitation	•	•	•
First-aid program	•	•	•
Flu shot program	•	•	•
Oral hygiene examination	•		•
Smoking cessation	•	•	•
Stress management		•	
Badminton			•
Basketball	•	•	
Karate	•	•	
Parent-tot swim	•	•	
Racquetball	•	•	
Scuba diving	•		
Social dance	•		
Tennis		•	
Yoga	•		

•Programs available at this site.

Emerson Hospital employees are allowed to use the Sentry facility during the work week if they have participated in the cardiovascular conditioning program. Recently, Sentry and the hospital started another joint program, Active Weight Loss. With two nutritionists from Emerson Hospital and an exercise specialist from Sentry, the program combines nutritional information, behavior modification, and learning to exercise properly. This cooperative effort has been extremely successful since its inception during the summer of 1980.

The subject of compliance and adherence to exercise is a question of great concern. The literature suggests dropout rates vary widely from 30% to 70% [8]. Michael Sachs addresses this issue in greater detail in chapter 3. Statistics are currently being gathered at Sentry. In all facilities, compliance has improved with each year.

In conclusion, the mortality rate of cardiovascular disease and stroke is now on the decline. There has been a decrease in per capita consumption of tobacco and saturated fats as well as better overall control of hypertension [10]. While exercise alone is not a panacea, taken together with the other dietary and behavior modification programs offered at Sentry, exercise is a significant factor in enhancing employees' health.

References

1. American College of Sports Medicine. *Guidelines for Graded Exercise Testing and Prescription.* 2nd ed. Philadelphia: Lea and Febiger, 1980.

2. Cantu, Robert C. *Toward Fitness.* New York: Human Sciences Press, 1980.

3. Freeland, M., Calat, G., and Schendler, C.E. Projections for national health expenditures 1980, 1985, 1990. *Health Care Financing Review,* 1:1–27, 1980.

4. Kolutak, R. Doctors try scare tactics to save patients' lives. *Chicago Tribune,* 30 April 1976, p. 6.

5. McNerney, W.J. A new direction for our medical system. *U.S. News and World Report,* 28 March 1977, pp. 39–45.

6. Pollock, M.L., Wilmore, J.H., and Fox, S.M. *Health and Fitness Through Physical Activity.* New York: John Wiley and Sons, 1978.

7. Public Health Service. *Forward Plan for 1977–1981.* Washington, D.C.: DHEW. p. 108

8. Sachs, M.L. Compliance and addiction to exercise. Presented to New England chapter of the American College of Sports Medicine. Danvers, Ma. November, 1980.

9. U.S. Department of Commerce, Bureau of Census. Health and nutrition. In *Statistical Abstract of the United States 1979.* Washington, D.C.: U.S. Government Printing Office.

10. Walker, W.J. Changing U.S. lifestyle and declining vascular mortality: Cause or coincidence? (editorial). *N. Engl. J. Med.* 297:163–165, 1977.

5 Commercial Fitness Centers

David Camaione, Ph.D.,
and
Gary Klencheski, M.S.

Cardio-Fitness Center

The concept of cardiovascular fitness is not new in the fitness industry; in fact a number of these private fitness centers exist in New York City to serve the corporate community. The development of a privately owned commercial cardiovascular fitness center in downtown Hartford, Connecticut (Cardio-Fitness Center) was intended to draw upon the numerous corporate businesses located in the insurance capital of the world. Over 20,000 executive-type personnel work in the areas surrounding the downtown section. Major corporations in the area include United Technologies, Pratt-Whitney Aircraft, Otis Elevator, Heublin, Travelers, Aetna Life and Casualty, the Hartford Insurance Group, Merrill-Lynch, Phoenix Mutual, and the seat of state government to name a few. The cardiovascular fitness center hoped to draw approximately 5% to 10% of these executive-type personnel or about 1,500.

The marketing presentation before corporate management stressed those benefits which the center could offer to executive-type employees. By providing a fitness facility with a scientifically based program, professional staff, and highly trained exercise specialists using the most up-to-date equipment and conditioning principles, the center could offer participants the means to an improved cardiovascular-respiratory system, improved muscular strength and endurance, and proper weight control. Significant improvement in a number of modifiable coronary risk factors would be possible, if participants followed the exercise program.

Several practical considerations also received careful planning. Convenience for members was a prime concern. The entrance of the building, therefore, is located within a ten-minute walk from most major corporations. The complex also includes an attached parking garage, one of Hartford's leading restaurants, and a major branch bank.

The facility is aesthetically well designed with wall-to-wall carpeting and full-length windows from floor to ceiling on two sides. It has a striking view from the third floor looking out into the Hartford community with the beautiful state capitol in the background. The facility possesses all universal variable-resistance weight equipment, treadmills, and bicycle ergometers for cardiovascular work.

A prospective member discusses the program with the professional staff who explain the benefits, services, and medical clearance. All members must have their personal physicians prescribe an exercise stress test and blood analysis. The results of these tests are returned to the physician who fills out an appropriate medical review form that provides the center with all the necessary information for programming the participant's exercise prescription. When this step is completed, the member is called in for orientation sessions.

During the first orientation session, the new member is taken into the physical assessment room, and the assistant director administers a number of tests. Four skinfold sites for body composition are taken. There is a demonstration of how blood pressure will be taken while the participant is riding on the bicycle ergometer; a sit-and-reach test for flexibility is administered. A staff member then fills out the cardiac risk factor profile form, and the member spends the remaining time with a registered dietitian who goes over the blood analysis information and gives information concerning diet and nutrition.

During the next orientation session, the members are weighed in the underwater weighing tank to determine body composition. It takes about 30 minutes to administer this text. Members have several options for the remaining time. They may use the equipment on the conditioning floor, take a sauna, or talk to the nutritionist if there wasn't time in the previous session.

For subsequent sessions, a ten-station circuit system is utilized for the conditioning sessions. The American College of Sports Medicine guidelines are followed for the frequency, duration, and intensity of workouts. The conditioning session is broken down into three parts: a warm-up phase, a workout phase, and a warm-down phase. The member's heartbeat is elevated slowly during the first stations, maintained at the proper intensity during the workout stations, and gradually returned downward during the warm-down stations. The ten-station circuit includes:

1. Warm-up (stretching, flexibility)
2. Rowing or arm flexion (muscular endurance)
3. Leg flexion or leg extension (muscular endurance)
4. Bench stepping or rope jumping (cardiovascular endurance)
5. Treadmills (cardiovascular endurance)
6. Bicycles (cardiovascular endurance)
7. Chest press or shoulder press (arm muscular endurance)
8. Hip flexion or sit-ups
9. Warm-down (walking with free weights)
10. Warm-down (stretching, flexibility)

Theoretically, appoximately 60 members can be handled at one time, since there are six pieces of equipment at each station. Each member must start at station one. The cardiovascular stations (stations 4,5,6) are in the middle of the circuit because it is important for participants to go from one cardio-vascular station to another in order to maintain their heart rates at the individually prescribed intensities. A perceived exertion chart is maintained; members are asked to rate their exertion at each of the cardiovascular stations.

The fitness facility is temperature and humidity controlled, and respec-tive locker rooms have a men's and a women's sauna. The lockers include small cubicles for securing the member's valuables, with ample space to hang the member's business suits on hangers between the lockers. At the end of each workout, the members must sign out just as they had to sign in.

Fitcorp

Fitcorp is a private corporation located at 133 Federal Street in Boston's business district. Incorporated in February 1979, Fitcorp's doors opened to the public in October 1979. Fitcorp occupies 14,000 square feet of space in the old Blue Cross-Blue Shield building.

Fitcorp is open Monday through Friday, between the hours of 7 a.m. and 7 p.m. The staff consists of five full-time professionals, four of whom are fitness professionals with either college or advanced degrees in exercise physiology or a related health enhancement field. Two staff people are certified by the American College of Sports Medicine as exercise test technicians.

The fitness center can accommodate a total of 800 men and women. At present, there are approximately 500 annual members. Fitcorp's chief objective is to serve the corporate community; at present, nearly half of the members receive some form of financial reimbursement from their place of business. Clients include some of Boston's leading banks, insurance compa-nies, brokerage houses, and private corporations.

Fitcorp's fee structure is based upon an annual individual membership fee of $395. A two-month trial membership for $95 can be applied toward the annual membership upon its expiration. To date, approximately 75% of the two-month members renew their memberships.

A membership entitles an individual to unlimited use of the Fitcorp facility and participation in any group program such as aerobic dance or slimnastics. Each member first receives a fitness evaluation for the purpose of collecting entry data to measure future progress or lack of it and develop-ing the individual exercise prescription. Most members exercise at Fitcorp on an individual basis.

A strong one-to-one relationship is developed by the staff with the members. All members are known on a first-name basis. Fitcorp's success can be attributed to three factors: first, the quality of programs and staff; second, the convenience of the location for members; and third, the attractiveness of the facility. Fitcorp neither looks nor smells like a gym.

University-Based Fitness Centers

Thomas Manfredi, Ph.D.
and
W. Jay Gillespie, Ed.D.

Exercise alone is not a rational approach toward lowering the morbidity and mortality of heart disease. Nutrition and diet counseling, smoking cessation programs, stress management counseling, and educational sessions dealing with topics such as cathartic and recreational aspects of exercise should be ancillary components of an exercise program. The rationale for this approach is based upon population studies such as the Minnesota studies [4] and the Multiple Risk Factor Invervention Trial study [3]. These studies appear to support the contention that life style and environmental factors can play a leading role in laying the foundation for cardiac disorders.

The University Setting

The availability of physical resources and academic expertise along with the potential for interdisciplinary approaches toward life-style enhancement afford the university environment a near ideal setting for an exercise program which emphasizes preventive health. Universities which have both physical education departments and medical schools have especially outstanding resources for developing sophisticated fitness programs. Usually the campus health care center can provide the necessary medical attention on campuses which do not have medical schools.

Some Basic Considerations of the University Setting

The biggest advantage of the university setting is the availability of outstanding exercise facilities which can be used, in most situations, at little or no cost. Facility overhead costs probably constitute the greatest proportion of a participant's cost for entering a fitness program which is administered in a privately owned facility.

Personnel costs at the university, in most cases, are minimal. Concomitant with this are the educational benefits which are passed on to the students who either volunteer or receive academic credit for staffing the program. Independent studies, honors theses, master's theses, and physiology courses have been structured around the adult fitness and cardiac rehabilitation programs at Southern Connecticut State College.

Low overhead cost for facilities and staffing offer the university an opportunity to charge minimal fees for enrollment. Furthermore, the physical education curriculum along with the large number of students available to the fitness program director not only afford the director an opportunity to enrich the students academically but also provide great resources for personnel selection.

Universities and corporations are finding that through concurring efforts adult fitness programs can be tailored to the specific needs and schedules of selected corporate personnel. In turn, corporations can provide monies to support primary and ancillary programs and purchase laboratory equipment which can further enhance the sophistication of the fitness program.

Prominent among the disadvantages of the college setting are the usual red tape problems associated with private, and especially nonprofit, institutions. Campus committees, campus administrators, the attorney general, the board, and possibly many other campus organizations must interact before unified action can be taken. These concerns coupled with the necessary medical community involvement provide administrative and political challenges to the program director, to say the least.

Another rather common problem associated with the university-based fitness program involves scheduling and sharing gymnasium and field house facilities. Physical education classes, athletic teams, and intramural programs which have been in existence as long as the universities themselves must often be imposed upon to cooperate with health-related fitness classes. Thus, any exercise physiologist who sets out to establish a university-based fitness program should possess not only the necessary academic expertise but also a knowledge of the basic administrative and political finesse which is necessary to deal successfully with the campus and community challenges.

Cosponsorship of Fitness Programs

Some university-based fitness programs are cosponsored with other nonprofit organizations. Southern Connecticut State College's Cardiac Rehabilitation Program, for example, is cosponsored with the South Central Chapter of the Connecticut Heart Association. This highly successful program provides a source of income for the Heart Association as well as monies for qualified graduate students at the college who run the exercise sessions, lecture to the patients, and attend the Heart Association committee meetings.

Southern Connecticut State College's program was constructed by Kevin Kear. Presently, a plan is in motion to employ the adult fitness program under a proposed Sports Medicine and Fitness Clinic at the college.

Typical University-Based Adult Fitness Program Personnel

The key personnel involved with the operation of a university-based fitness program should be a program director, a medical director, an exercise physiologist, and an executive board. The executive board can consist of a key campus administrator (dean, academic vice-president), a key faculty member (chairperson of physical education department), a cardiologist, an orthopedic physican or a physical therapist with expertise in sports medicine, a key corporate executive, a lawyer, and a community-minded politician.

Graduate and upper-class undergraduate students along with selected faculty members can play important roles as exercise leaders and lecturers. Coaches, physical therapists, and sports medicine physicians can provide the participants with very practical and stimulating mini-clinics (for example, basic orthopedic concerns of running).

Preliminary Screening of Participants

The preliminary screening of participants should be accomplished for the purpose of diagnosis, exercise prescription, and attainment of physiologic and orthopedic baseline data. The major components of the preliminary screening should be first, cardiodiagnostic screening consisting of a graded exercise test, selected blood chemistries, and a risk factor score [11] along with a physician's subjective appraisal of the participant; second, a body composition assessment utilizing appropriate population specific skinfold formulas [6] or underwater weighing techniques; and third, questionnaires relative to the participant's nutritional, exercise, and leisure habits. Whenever appropriate, proper consent and referral forms should be used [1,14].

The Graded Exercise Stress-Test Protocol

The graded exercise stress protocol is a very important part of the university-based fitness program. The objectives of the exercise stress test should be to: (1) assess physiologic performance in response to low, moderate, and high workloads; (2) prescribe exercise; and (3) provide baseline data for progress assessment.

An important advantage of the university setting is that a stress-testing laboratory offers the opportunity to conduct a graded exercise test under controlled conditions, assuming all participants are evaluated by the same team of clinicians utilizing the same instruments, methods, and procedures for establishing data. The brief discussion which follows serves to reinforce the importance of carefully controlled stress-testing protocol and reliable assessment of participant progress and program effectiveness.

Exercise prescription is quite often based upon a maximal heart rate value or predicted maximal MET level achieved while exercising on a treadmill or bicycle ergometer. While prescribing exercise based upon training heart rate has distinct advantages over METs [13], symptom-limited tests can occur in supposedly asymptomatic individuals. This situation more often occurs in older people. Wilmore [13] and Sidney and Shephard [10] present excellent discussions on exercise prescription and assessment of physiologic improvement in response to exercise.

Attempts to assess physiologic responses to training should not be limited to treadmill tests designed to measure or predict maximal aerobic capacity or maximal heart rate. Such tests may often be insensitive to a person's cardiopulmonary responses to stress at low or moderate intensities of effort.

When administering a graded exercise stress test, one should follow the guidelines established by the American College of Sports Medicine [1]. Heart rate, blood pressure, double product (HR × systolic BP/100), oxygen pulse (VO_2/heart beat), ventilation equivalent (VE/VO_2), and respiratory exchange ratio should each be assessed at all workloads during a graded exercise stress test. If each physiologic parameter is graphically plotted at low, moderate, and high workloads, oxygen pulse changes, for example, can provide valuable baseline data. The baseline graphs can later be compared to post-training graphs. A postprogram exercise stress test may, for example, show a less drastic rise in oxygen pulse at a moderate workload. This would indicate that the heart is pumping more oxygen per beat at moderate workloads as a result of training.

When a graded exercise stress-test protocol is followed as suggested above, the data obtained can be very sensitive to the specificity of response to exercises of different intensities, durations, frequencies, and modalities. In view of this, it is suggested that such tests be performed in the same laboratory on all participants in an effort to insure a carefully controlled setting. If a university-based fitness program is organized properly through coordinated efforts with the medical community, a common stress-testing laboratory will become an integral part of the program.

Noteworthy Resources of the University-Based Fitness Program

Perhaps the most salient resource available to the university setting is its diversified faculty. For example, most universities are capable of offering an adult fitness program which includes swimming, jogging, bicycling, aerobic dance, and racquetball. Each of these activities is aerobic and shows some specificity of training. The university setting has the faculty expertise and facilities to offer a few or all of these activities in a single 12- or 16-week fitness course. Such a course offers the participant experiences with different modalities of exercise training, which later provide him with a number of choices for future exercise activities.

All exercise programs should be supplemented with educational classes. Lecture topics such as the proper way to run, swim, or bicycle; common injuries and how to avoid them; warm-up and stretching techniques; and nutritional counseling are especially appropriate for people engaging in an exercise program for the first time.

As expressed earlier, fitness programs should be a part of an interdisciplinary approach to life-style enhancement on the premise that life-style enrichment and preventive health go hand in hand. Family counseling, diet and nutrition counseling, stress control, and recreation counseling can often enhance a participant's life style. Such programs are available or can be constructed at the university. When coordinated properly, these programs become ancillary resources to the fitness program and provide an effective approach toward life-style alteration and primary prevention of coronary heart disease.

The Cardiovascular Health and Exercise Center at Northeastern University

One of the aims of the Cardiovascular Health and Exercise Center at Northeastern University is to investigate the role of exercise in cardiovascular health and disease. Growing evidence suggests that life-style changes in the quality and quantity of exercise, improved nutritional practices (for example, decreasing consumption of fats, cholesterol, and salt while increasing consumption of complex carbohydrates), weight reduction, smoking cessation, and stress management can reduce the risk of cardiovascular disease and help in the rehabilitation of those with cardiovascular disease.

A second aim of the center is to provide service. The center provides cardiovascular disease prevention, intervention, and rehabilitation programs designed to serve the greater Boston business and medical communities. As Americans become more active and health conscious, the need increases for programs of medical testing and evaluation, exercise prescription and supervised exercise, and health education to guide people through the initial stages of an exercise program. A safe, enjoyable, and fruitful experience encourages a lifelong commitment to keeping fit and staying healthy. A medically supervised, scientifically structured program is critically important for people who are past the age of 35, who may possess one or more coronary-risk factors, who have documented coronary artery disease, who have suffered a myocardial infarction, or who have undergone coronary bypass or valvular surgery.

The third aim of the center is to provide for a segment of the education of health and exercise professionals. On-campus programs, as well as programs conducted at off-campus sites at companies and public school gymnasia provide laboratories which enable undergraduate and graduate students in physical education, physical therapy, nursing, and health education to gain firsthand experience as preventive/rehabilitative exercise technologists, exercise specialists, health counselors, teachers, physical therapists, and researchers.

Administration

The Northeastern University Cardiovascular Health and Exercise Center is administered through the physical education department of Boston-Bouvé College of Human Development Professions, one of eight basic colleges of the university. Northeastern University is the largest private institution of higher learning in the country with an enrollment totalling approximately 45,000 students. Table 6-1 indicates the composition of the center's staff and medical advisory committee.

Programs

The center provides programs for cardiovascular disease prevention, intervention, and rehabilitation and for promotion of improved cardiovascular health of all, regardless of the individual's current health status. Each program includes:

1. A cardiovascular medical evaluation, a graded exercise test, pulmonary function testing, body composition assessments, blood analysis, psychological testing, physical fitness testing, and coronary risk factor screening and evaluation at intake, during, and upon program completion.

Table 6-1
Staff and Medical Advisory Committee of the Northeastern University Cardiovascular Health and Exercise Center

Name	Position/Affiliation
Staff	
W. Jay Gillespie, Ed.D.	Director Exercise physiologist Associate professor of physical education
Michael D. Klein, M.D.	Cardiologist Medical director
Catherine Certo, M.S., R.P.T.	Cardiopulmonary physical therapist Assistant professor of physical therapy Coordinator, Cardiac Rehabilitation Program
Elizabeth Eagan-Bengston, M.S.	Preventive/rehabilitative exercise specialist Administrative assistant Coordinator of the exercise physiology laboratory
Pamela Drummond, B.S., R.N.	Cardiac rehabilitation nurse specialist Coordinator of patient education
Delaine Williamson, M.S., R.N., R.D.	Nutrionist and lecturer
—	Graduate teaching assistants (2)
—	Preventive/rehabilitative exercise technologists (6)
—	Exercise leaders (6)
Medical Advisory Committee	
Sidney Alexander, M.D.	Head, Cardiovascular Section Lahey Clinic Medical Center
Charlotte Crockett	American Heart Association
Saul Cohen, M.D.	Director, Health Care Associates
Job E. Fuchs, M.D.	Director, Lane Health Center, Northeastern University
Robert Habasevich, R.P.T., M.S.	Director of Rehabilitation Services, Affiliate Hospital Center, Inc.
L. Howard Hartley, M.D.	Department of Cardiology, Massachusetts General Hospital Associate Professor of Medicine, Harvard Medical School
John Markis, M.D.	Department of Cardiology, Beth Israel Hospital
Lyle J. Micheli, M.D.	Director, Division of Sports Medicine, Children's Hospital Medical Center
Stuart Soeldner, M.D.	Joslin Research Laboratories
Michael D. Klein, M.D.	Chairman

2. Prescribed and supervised exercise classes in jogging, aerobic dance, aerobic swimming, and competitive running.
3. Health education seminars on coronary risk reduction.
4. Individual counseling in nutrition, weight reduction, smoking termination, and stress management for those in need.

These programs are designed to serve the following groups of people:

1. The apparently healthy, asymptomatic, sedentary adult past the age of 35 with additional risk factors and individuals of any age with multiple risk factors and who are found to be at moderate to high risk are candidates for the preventive health program. The program is not for people below the age of 35 who are physically active on a regular basis and at below moderate risk.
2. Asymptomatic individuals with multiple risk factors, individuals with positive graded exercise test results (ischemia and severe arrhythmias) and symptomatic individuals who are judged to be at high risk and are candidates for the cardiac intervention program.
3. Individuals who are a minimum of six to eight weeks after myocardial infarction or bypass and valvular surgery are placed in the cardiac rehabilitation program.

The sources of participants for the three programs include the following:

1. Employees of Northeastern University are candidates for programs conducted on the Boston campus.
2. Students attending University College (part-time, evening division), Northeastern University, enroll in programs presently conducted on the Boston and Burlington campuses.
3. Employees of major corporations such as the Gillette Company and the Polaroid Corporation enroll in programs conducted on the Boston campus and at the company's site provided the company has the facilities.
4. Employees of small firms located in Boston's Back Bay and Prudential Center areas are close to Northeastern's campus.
5. Residents of the area surrounding the Boston and Burlington campuses.
6. Cardiac patients referred from physicians and outpatient programs in hospitals in the greater Boston area are eligible for the cardiac rehabilitation program.

The Preventive Health Programs

The programs that emphasize cardiovascular disease prevention and health promotion begin with a cardiovascular medical and physical fitness evaluation for all participants. Some elect to take this evaluation only and utilize the results for their own purposes in consultation with their physicians. Most participants, however, enroll in a complete course in cardiovascular health and exercise which includes the medical evaluation at intake, three months of thrice weekly exercise classes, weekly health seminars in coronary risk reduction, and a reevaluation at the completion of the three months to measure progress. Graduates of the course or those completing just the evaluation are eligible to participate in the fitness maintenance programs which include a jogging club and courses in aerobic swimming, aerobic dance, and competitive running. For executive groups of between 6 to 12 there is the executive stress-management program. After completing the three-month course in cardiovascular health and exercise, these groups participate in an extended nine-day experience of camping, canoeing, and climbing in the wilderness for the purposes of team building and individual stress management.

Cardiovascular Medical and Physical Fitness Evaluation. Although some symptoms of coronary artery disease, such as angina pectoris, are often apparent in the heart disease victim, approximately 20% to 30% of all sudden deaths were not preceded by any reported symptoms by the victims. In fact, there are very few noninvasive clinical methods used in the initial diagnosis of this hidden killer.

In addition to angina, there are certain changes on both the resting and exercise electrocardiogram (ECG) and alterations in serum enzyme concentrations suggestive of either an impending or previous myocardial infarction.

However, an individual's relative risk of suffering a myocardial infarction can be estimated by identifying a variety of health factors that have been statistically linked with the development of coronary artery disease. These coronary risk factors include hypertension, hyperlipidemia, cigarette smoking, family history of heart disease, diabetes, obesity, physical inactivity, stress, type A personality, and certain ECG abnormalities. Before one begins a program of preventive health which includes exercise, these coronary risk factors must be identified and evaluated. This is particularly critical for the sedentary male past the age of 35 who may possess any one or more of the risk factors.

This test battery is designed to evaluate the individual's cardiovascular health status, identify and evaluate his coronary risk profile, evaluate his functional capacity and physical fitness, and provide guidelines for establishing the initial exercise prescription. The evaluation begins with a detailed review of the participant's present, past, and family medical history including a survey of nutritional, smoking, drinking, and exercise habits. This is accomplished via a written questionnaire completed by the participant prior to his test date. In addition, participants who have a personal physician are required to obtain their physician's consent by having their physician complete a physician's referral form which includes basic medical data obtained from his most recent physical exam (not to exceed one year). On the day of the tests the participant is given an informed consent form which he reads and signs in the presence of a witness.

Next, a sample of blood is drawn from the participant. A complete blood count, hemoglobin, and hematocrit is routinely done to determine an individual's oxygen-carrying capacity of the blood and to screen for the presence of anemia or polycythemia. If the white cell count is outside the normal range, a differential count is performed. Cholesterol, high density lipoprotein, triglycerides, glucose, and serum enzymes are obtained from the SMA 25 results, and a lipid profile is developed and evaluated on the basis of normative data.

Percent body fat and lean body weight are estimated from obtaining present body weight and four skinfold measurements (triceps, biceps, subscapular, and suprailiac) and utilizing the regression equations developed by Durnin and Wormesley. The percent body fat is then evaluated on the basis of normative data. From these data an ideal percent fat is chosen, and an ideal weight and projected weight loss is then calculated.

Vital capacity and forced expiratory volume in one second are obtained on a respirator. The results are used to screen for the presence of pulmonary obstruction diseases (asthma, bronchitis, emphysema, and so forth) which will limit functional capacity and improvement in cardiovascular endurance. A cardiopulmonary examination is conducted by a cardiologist prior to the graded exercise test.

The graded exercise test is conducted on a motor-driven treadmill according to either the Bruce, Balke, or Wilmore protocols depending upon the age, health status, and estimated functional capacity of the participants. A 12-lead ECG and blood pressure is obtained prior to exercise (supine, standing, and after 20 seconds of hyperventilation), at the completion of each stage of the exercise protocol, and at two minute intervals of a walking recovery for six minutes or until the heart rate is less than 100 beats per minute. Participants are encouraged to exercise to voluntary maximal exertion or until their heart rate equals or exceeds the age-projected maximum heart rate. Maximal oxygen uptake is predicted from the treadmill speed and elevation, and the functional capacity is then evaluated on the basis of normative data. The heart rates and blood pressures obtained at each stage of the exercise test are plotted on a graph, and the hemodynamic response to exercise is evaluated. The 12-lead ECG's are evaluated by the cardiologist for changes suggestive of ischemia and the presence of arrhythmias.

Maximal oxygen uptake as well as minute ventilation, frequency of ventilation, tidal volume, respiratory exchange rates, and METS can be obtained directly with the use of an automated metabolic and pulmonary measurement system. This is an option that is used for selected patients for research purposes or upon request. It is not used routinely for everyone.

Low back dysfunction is a prevalent problem among the adult population and is chiefly due to tight, inflexible low back muscles and weak abdominal muscles causing a forward tilting pelvic girdle and increased lordosis. Flexibility of the low back extensor muscles and hip extensors is evaluated with a sit and reach test. Abdominal muscle strength and endurance is evaluated by the maximum number of sit-ups the person can perform in one minute. Overall body strength is grossly estimated from grip strength obtained with a grip dynamometer.

Three personality and behavorial inventories are administered in a comfortable conference room following the individual's taking a shower and changing back into street clothes. The results from these tests are used to evaluate certain personality traits and stress-related moods that are associated with coronary artery disease. Aspects of the California Psychological Inventory are used to measure the traits of sociability, self-control, achievement, and flexibility. The Jenkins Activity Survey assesses type A personality traits in a composite score as well as the components of speed and impatience, job involvement, and hard driving scores. The profile of mood states measures the six stress-related mood states of tension and anxiety, depression, anger and hostility, vigor, fatigue, and confusion.

The results of the cardiovascular medical and physical fitness evaluation are presented to the participant and to the referring physician via a computer generated three-page report which includes an evaluation of all scores (percentage of body fat, blood lipids, blood pressures, heart rate, maximal oxygen uptake, pulmonary function, and pulmonary function tests) on the basis of age group norms, a graph of heart rate and blood pressure response to the graded exercise test, ECG interpretation, and a coronary risk profile. The results are further interpreted to the individual in a two-hour lecture approximately five days after testing and in individual consultation with the physician if warranted.

All testing is conducted in the Exercise Physiology Laboratory at Northeastern's Boston campus. The complete test battery requires two and one-half to three hours to complete.

Cardiovascular Health and Exercise Course. A complete course in cardiovascular health and exercise is offered for the apparently healthy, but sedentary, adult past 35 years of age. This beginning course (number 62.410) in exercise and preventive health provides three-quarter hours of academic credit and is offered through Northeastern's University College (part-time, evening division). Participants may choose to receive a letter grade, a pass-fail grade, or to audit the course.

The course includes:

1. The complete cardiovascular medical and physical fitness evaluation described previously
2. Three months of supervised exercise classes conducted three times a week
3. Ten weekly health education seminars in coronary risk reduction with accompanying testbooks and handouts
4. Complete locker room accommodations and use of indoor running track or gymnasium and available parking
5. The complete cardiovascular medical and physical fitness evaluation, readministered at the completion of the course to measure improvement

Exercise Classes. Each one-hour exercise class includes 15 minutes of warm-up exercises, 20 to 40 minutes of jogging at a prescribed intensity and duration, and 10 minutes of warm-down exercises. Each participant's exercise program is individually prescribed, based on the initial evaluation results.

The initial exercise prescription is set according to the American College of Sports Medicine guidelines recommendations. The exercise intensity is set to between 70% to 85% of the person's maximum heart rate obtained on the graded exercise test. Individuals begin exercising with their heart rate within this target zone for 2-minute work intervals with 1-minute recovery intervals alternated to total 30 minutes of intermittent exercise. Progression is applied from this base by increasing the duration of each work interval and decreasing the number of recovery intervals until the prescribed intensity can be sustained for 30 to 40 minutes in duration. Classes meet at a frequency of three times per week (Monday, Wednesday, and Friday), and participants are encouraged to engage in a fourth session on the weekend when they become reconditioned.

Exercise is directed by exercise specialists who continuously monitor each individual's exercise prescription. The exercise specialist-to-participant ratio is no greater than one to six in order to ensure individual attention. Bicycle ergometers and treadmills are available for anyone for whom jogging is inadvisable.

Health Seminars. Weekly health-education seminars in coronary risk reduction provide assistance to individuals who plan a lifelong commitment to exercise and improved health behavior. Discussions, conducted by faculty, focus on topics such as:

1. Coronary artery disease and its risk factors
2. Role of exercise in cardiovascular health and disease
3. Nutrition and cardiovascular health (two weeks)
4. Diet and weight reduction (two weeks)
5. Stress, personality type, and cardiovascular health (two weeks)
6. Stress management and relaxation techniques
7. Smoking cessation

Exercise classes are conducted throughout the year on the Boston campus, Monday, Wednesday, and Friday from 7:30 a.m. to 8:30 a.m., with an additional section from 5:00 p.m. to 6:00 p.m. in April through September. On the Burlington campus, classes are between 4:30 p.m. to 6:30 p.m. (two sections) on Monday, Wednesday, and Friday. Health seminars are conducted on Wednesdays from 7:30 a.m. to 8:30 a.m. in Boston and at 6:00 p.m. in Burlington.

Fitness Maintenance Programs

Jogging Club. The purpose of the Jogging Club is to provide a structured exercise program for people completing the cardiovascular health and exercise course. Although some people can develop an exercise habit within three months; six months to a year in a structured and disciplined program are necessary for most people to become sufficiently motivated to continue regular exercise as a way of life.

As an incentive, the Jogging Club offers awards for joggers who accumulate 50, 100, 250, 500, 750, and 1,000 running miles. In addition, members' names and accumulated mileage are published in the club's quarterly newsletter, *Cardiovascular Lifelines*. Members can choose to participate in from 9 to 12 sessions a week in structured warm-ups conducted by exercise leaders, and they have the use of exercise rooms, the indoor running track, lockers, and the shower facilities located in the Cabot Physical Education Center.

The Road Runners is a branch of the club for members entering competitive road races. Social events, conducted annually by the club's social committee, include a spring Fun Run, a fall tasting party, and an awards banquet.

Membership is open to graduates of the cardiovascular health and exercise course. Full membership includes participation in the mileage club, subscription to *Cardiovascular Lifelines*, participation in structured warm-up classes, and use of the Cabot locker room and indoor running track. Associate membership includes participation in the mileage club and subscription to *Cardiovascular Lifelines*. No facilities privileges are included.

Competitive Running Course. Training and racing techniques, and nutritional practices are discussed in the competitive running course. Participants compete in 2.5-, 5.0-, and 6.2-mile road races, conducted every weekend in the greater Boston area. In conjunction with Jogging Club hours, classes meet three times a week during the fall and spring. Completion of the cardiovascular health and exercise course or the cardiovascular medical and physical fitness evaluation is a prerequisite for this course.

Aerobic Dance Course. Choreographed exercise and dance movements to popular rock, disco, and classical music are designed to produce an aerobic-training effect and to develop cardiovascular endurance, as well as muscular endurance, muscle tone, improved posture, and flexibility. Classes meet Tuesdays and Thursdays at noon during winter and spring. Completion of the cardiovascular health and exercise course or cardiovascular medical and physical fitness evaluation is a prerequisite for this course.

Aerobic Swimming Course. Continuous, rhythmical swimming, accompanied by music, is designed to develop cardiovascular endurance and provide an aerobic-training effect. Students should have acquired beginning-level skills in the elementary backstroke, breast stroke, and freestyle stroke prior to enrolling. Classes meet Tuesdays and Thursdays at 7:00 a.m. during the summer and fall. Completion of the cardiovascular health and exercise course or the cardiovascular medical and physical fitness evaluation is a prerequisite for this course.

Executive Stress-Management Program

The Executive Stress-Management Program is designed for groups of 6 to 12 executives who are employed by the same corporation and who function as a team in their organization. The purpose of this program is to build a more efficient team and to develop individual stress-management skills during eight days of physical challenges in the wilderness. Prior to the wilderness experience, participants receive physical fitness testing, behavior testing, and three months of physical fitness training. A one-day artificial challenge course and instruction in basic canoeing skills are segments of the preparation. The program includes:

1. The complete cardiovascular medical and physical fitness evaluation described previously
2. The three-month cardiovascular health and exercise course
3. A one-day program, conducted at Northeastern University's Warren Center, Ashland, Massachusetts, with a series of challenges on a ropes course constructed in nearby woods, and basic canoeing skills
4. Eight days of camping, canoeing, and mountain climbing in the Allagash wilderness in Maine
5. A three-month program to maintain fitness and establish a personal exercise regimen that can continue beyond the program

The Wilderness Experience. An eight-day outdoor experience provides the complexity of a real-life situation in which participants develop stress-identifying skills and coping techniques, without the immediate pressure associated with an on-the-job location. Participants canoe from the Northeast Carry on the west branch of the Penobscot River to Lake Chesundook and Lake Umbazooksus. A two-mile portage to Mud Pond then leads to Chamberlain Lake and further canoeing through Churchill Lake, down the Allagash River to Allagash Village. A canoe-run down Chase Rapids and some mountain climbing constitute additional stress experiences to be confronted during the trip.

Discussions preceding each stress experience focus on specific stress situations to be anticipated and help to envision appropriate stress-management responses. After each experience, discussions provide relevant feedback, based on the participants' confrontation of the situation. The discussions also help to correlate these stress situations with those that occur in the work environment and draw parallels between the techniques for managing stress in each circumstance. Participants are encouraged to develop and implement the same techniques for stress management that can be practiced effectively in an office environment.

The field experience is not structured to be a wilderness, minimum-survival test. With the exception of appropriate clothing and a sleeping bag, participants are provided with all necessary equipment for the trip, including tents and plenty of nutritious food, as well as all travel arrangements.

Benefits of Preventive Health Programs

Preventive health programs can improve an individual's physical fitness by increasing functional capacity (maximal oxygen uptake), decreasing resting and submaximal exercise heart rates and blood pressures, and increasing the heart's stroke volume. Body weight and percentage of body fat can also be reduced, especially if exercise is combined with proper diet. Increased physical activity and decreased body fat can significantly decrease serum triglycerides and cholesterol and can increase high density lipoproteins, all of which reduce coronary risk. Stress-related behaviors such as tension, anxiety, depression, anger, hostility, and fatigue can be exchanged for vigor, alertness, and joie de vivre. Certain personality characteristics (speed and impatience, high job involvement, and hard driving motivation) associated with increased risk such as the composite type A personality may be modified as people learn to more effectively handle stress. Additionally, people who receive regular stimulation from exercise seek it less often from nicotine, caffeine, and alcohol.

In addition to benefitting individuals, these programs can benefit organizations. Similar programs have been shown to improve employee morale, efficiency, and productivity. Absenteeism and extended losses due to hospitalization and disability may be decreased with improved employee health and fitness. Group health and life insurance premiums may decrease as a result of demonstrating a reduction in paid benefits. These considerations are important in view of recent statistics released by the American Association of Fitness Directors in Business and Industry. According to that group, coronary disease results in $3 billion per year in direct costs, $28 billion in indirect costs from death and disability, and 130 million lost workdays annually.

References

1. American College of Sports Medicine. *Guidelines for Graded Exercise Testing and Exercise Prescription.* Philadelphia: Lea and Febiger, 1980.

2. American College of Sports Medicine. Policy statement regarding the use of human subjects and informed consent. *Med. Sci. Sports Exercise* 12:1, 1980.

3. Benfari, R.C. Lifestyle alteration and the primary prevention of CHD: The Multiple Risk Factor Intervention Trial (MRFIT). In M.L. Pollock, D.H. Schmidt, and D.T. Mason (Eds.), *Heart Disease and Rehabilitation.* Boston: Houghton Mifflin Publishers, 1979, Pp. 341-351.

4. Blackburn, H. Preventive cardiology in practice: Minnesota studies on risk factor reduction. In M.L. Pollock, D.H. Schmidt, and D.T. Mason (Eds.), *Heart Disease and Rehabilitation.* Boston: Houghton Mifflin Publishers, 1979, Pp. 245-275.

5. Gilliam, T.B., Katch, V.L., Thorland, W., and Weltman, A. Prevalence of coronary heart disease risk factors in active children 7 to 12 years of age. *Med. Sci. Sports* 9:1 21-25, 1977.

6. Jackson, A.S., and Pollock, M.L. Prediction accuracy of body density, lean body weight, and total body volume equations. *Med. Sci. Sports* 9:4, 197–201, 1977.

7. Morris, J.N., Heady, J.A., Raffle, P.A.B., Roberts, C.G., and Parks, J.W. Coronary heart disease and physical activity of work. *Lancet* 2:1053–1111, 1953.

8. New York Academy of Sciences (Ed.). The Marathon: Physiological, Medical, Epidemiological Studies. *Annals of the New York Academy of Sciences,* 1977, p. 346.

9. Rosenmann, R.H., Brand, R.J., Sholtz, R.I., and Friedman, M. Multivariate prediction of coronary heart disease during 8.5 year follow-up in the Western Collaborative Group study. *Am. J. Cardiol.* 37:903–910, 1976.

10. Sidney, K.H., and Shepard, R.J. Frequency and intensity of exercise training for elderly subjects. *Med. Sci. Sports* 10:2, 125–131, 1978.

11. Stamler, J. Research related to risk factors. *Circulation* 60:7, 1575–1587, 1979.

12. Truett, J., Cornfield, J., and Kannel, W. A multivariate analysis of the risk of coronary heart disease in Framingham. *J. Chronic Dis.* 20:511–524, 1967.

13. Wilmore, J.H. Applied physiologic concerns and benefits in cardiac rehabilitation. In M.L. Pollock, D.H. Schmidt, and D.T. Mason (Eds.), *Heart Disease and Rehabilitation.* Boston: Houghton Mifflin Publishers, 1979, Pp. 678–689.

14. Wilson, P.K., Winga, E.R., Edgett, J.W., and Gushiken, T.T. *Policies and Procedures of a Cardiac Rehabilitation Program.* Philadelphia: Lea and Febiger, 1978.

15. Wood, P.D., Haskell, W., Klein, H., Lewis, S., Stern, M.P., and Farquhar, J.W. The distribution of plasma lipoproteins in middle-aged male runners. *Metabolism* 25:11, 1249–1256, 1976.

Special Considerations
for the Exercising Adult

7 Nutrition and Human Performance

National Dairy Council

Within the past several years there has been a promising resurgence of interest in physical performance [1]. According to a 1977 Gallup Poll almost half of American adults exercise regularly to keep fit. Tennis, bicycling, swimming, calisthenics, walking, and running are among some of the more popular forms of exercise [1]. For persons engaged in normal activities or light to moderate exercise, for athletes who train and compete, for military recruits, and for those in occupations such as mining or heavy construction, nutrition is an important, although certainly not the only factor affecting the individual's overall physical performance [2].

As reviewed in a previous *Dairy Council Digest* [3] and supported by most authorities [4–15], a nutritionally balanced diet based on the four food groups with sufficient calories to meet energy demands will satisfy all the nutritional requirements of most active persons. For those involved in activities of high intensity or prolonged duration (for example, distance running) special nutritional needs appear to be indicated [2,13,16,17]. Such needs can be met by modifying the diet, as opposed to ingestion of special ergogenic work-producing dietary aids which may prove detrimental. This chapter reviews some of the more recent findings and recommendations regarding dietary intake in relation to physical performance.

Diet Guidelines

The Basic Diet

The diet that will provide the best performance for athletes must contain adequate quantities of water, energy, protein, fat, carbohydrate, vitamins,

Reproduced with permission from the *Dairy Council Digest* 51:13–17, 1980. Copyright © 1980 by National Dairy Council. The summary from page 13 of the original article has been omitted. National Dairy Council assumes the responsibility for writing and editing this article. However, the help and suggestions of the following reviewers are acknowledged: D.L. Costill, Ph.D., professor and director, Human Performance Laboratory, Ball State University, Muncie, Indiana; N.J. Smith, M.D., professor, Department of Pediatrics and Sports Medicine, University of Washington, Seattle, Washington; and D.S. Wiggans, Ph.D., professor, Department of Biochemistry, University of Texas, Southwestern Medical School, Dallas, Texas.

minerals, and electrolytes in suitable proportions [3]. A nutritionally balanced diet not too dissimilar from what the average American eats each day is recommended [14,18]. According to the results of a U.S. household food consumption survey conducted in the spring of 1977, 14% of food energy was supplied by protein, 43% by fat, and 42% by carbohydrate [19]. For athletes in training, greater emphasis is given to carbohydrates, with dietary energy derived as follows: 10% to 20% protein, 30% to 35% fat, and 50% to 55% carbohydrate [14,20]. And for athletes who train exhaustively on successive days and/or compete in prolonged endurance events, a diet containing more than 70% carbohydrate has proven beneficial to enhance performance [4,6].

More so in the past [4] but even recently [20], large amounts of protein have been considered necessary to improve performance, hence the popularity of highly promoted protein formulations of various types. Fifty-one percent of 75 coaches and trainers recently surveyed believed that protein was the most important factor to increase muscle mass [21]. This misconception has been difficult to dissipate. Muscle mass can be increased only by appropriate exercise. The weight of scientific data suggests that muscular activity does not increase the body's need for protein (0.8 grams per kilogram body weight/day) beyond the amount consumed in a normal diet [4,5]. A diet containing as much as 2.8 grams protein per kilogram body weight does not enhance physiological work performance during intensive physical training [22]. Furthermore, contraindications to a high-protein diet include possible ketosis, dehydration, and hyperuricemia with the threat of gout [3,18,20]. Protein, while essential to build and repair tissues, is the least important nutrient as an energy source [4,20,23].

Results of early analyses of respiratory exchange ratios and more recent sensitive analytical methods substantiate that both fat and carbohydrate are the major fuels for muscular activity [4,16,23–29]. The metabolism of fat and carbohydrates (and to a minor degree, proteins) generate adenosine triphosphate (ATP) which is the ultimate source of energy for working muscle cells. The relative contribution of each of these fuels depends on the duration and intensity of work, the individual's total work capacity or maximal oxygen uptake (VO_2 max), and diet. Fat (triglycerides in muscle cells and free fatty acids derived from triglycerides stored in adipose tissue) is the primary fuel for muscle activity in mild to moderate aerobic activities (for example, walking at 20% to 30% VO_2 max). As performance increases in intensity (70% VO_2 max) and oxygen availability to the working muscle becomes more limited, the body's fuel supply switches to more carbohydrate (muscle and liver glycogen and blood glucose). Less oxygen is required to metabolize carbohydrate than fat [4]. If submaximal (aerobic) work continues in duration, fat becomes a prevalent fuel source; during sustained high level activity, carbohydrate utilization is greatly increased [4].

Because fat is a less readily-available source of energy, and it has almost unlimited storage in the body, there is no rationale for increasing the fat content of the diet. In fact, high-fat diets, by creating a condition of acidosis, adversely affect performance [4,6]. On the other hand, carbohydrate, stored as glycogen in muscle and liver, can become depleted during repeated bursts of intense activity (for example, sprinting) or during long, exhaustive exercise (for example, distance running, cross-country skiing). Strauzenberg et al. [25] have shown that when glycogen falls below 5 grams per kilogram wet muscle, efficiency and performance rapidly deteriorate. Thus, the length of time an athlete can sustain physical work of high intensity depends in part on the content of muscle glycogen [16,25–29]. In terms of diet, it has been repeatedly demonstrated that inclusion of carbohydrate in the diet increases utilization of blood glucose, storage of muscle and liver glycogen, and ultimately endurance performance [16,27–29]. Conversely, a low-carbohydrate diet (that is, fad weight-reducing regimens) would, by leading to depletion of carbohydrate in muscles and liver, render it difficult for the individual to participate in vigorous physical activities or training [4].

As energy expenditure is increased by work, physical exercise, and athletic performance, the quantity of the basic diet consumed should be compatible with maintaining an efficient body weight and meeting the increased energy requirements of the activity [4,6,20]. Excess body fat decreases mechanical work efficiency; that is, more energy and oxygen are required to produce a given amount of physical work [8]. For highly-trained male athletes in top condition, the ideal fat content for some sports is 5% to 8% of body weight; for females it is 9% to 10% [20]. This compares with a fat content of 10% to 15% body weight in well-nourished nonathletic males and 20% to 25% in females [14].

Several factors influence the energy cost of exercise. These include the individual's age, sex, size (body weight and height), and metabolic rate, and the type, intensity, frequency, and duration of the activity [6]. For example, a heavier person expends more energy than a lighter-weight person for a given activity, and the energy cost of short-distance racing is less than marathon races [4,6,30]. Energy turnover among athletes varies from about 3,000 to 5,000 kilocalories daily, increasing an additional 500 to 1,500 kilocalories during training [14]. Normally, appetite and satiety are sensitive regulators automatically adjusting energy intake to meet the increased energy requirements [4,6,8,14,20]. However, under the emotional stress of training and competition, the athlete may fail to consume sufficient energy or alternatively, eat excessively. The increased energy demands should be accommodated by greater intake of high quality carbohydrate foods (for example, enriched grain products).

Body fluid balance is of utmost importance in attaining maximal physical performance [4,5,13,15–17,31–34]. Dehydration is one of the major limiting factors in physical work capacity. Water requirements are significantly increased under conditions of heavy work in warm environments. When more than 2% to 3% of the body's weight is acutely lost by exercise-induced sweating, circulatory and thermoregulatory functions are diminished [4,5,8,13,32]. Individuals who have low fitness levels and who are not acclimatized to the environmental heat tolerate fluid losses less well than athletes in better condition. Dehydration, by decreasing blood volume, limits the circulatory system's capacity to transport blood to the skin where body heat can be dissipated and to the working muscles where essential nutrients are needed. In severe cases this can lead to heat exhaustion and even death. The need for adequate fluid replenishment before, during, and after physical performance cannot be overemphasized. There is no basis for restricting water intake of athletes. In fact, the American College of Sports Medicine, recognizing the dangers of dehydration, published a position paper on this very subject, outlining guidelines to prevent heat injuries during distance running [34].

Although sweat loss can be substantial, the loss of electrolytes and minerals in sweat is relatively small [16]. A bodyweight loss of 5.8% by dehydration can decrease total exchangeable sodium and chloride by 6% to 8%, and potassium and magnesium by about 1% [13,16]. Renal conservation of electrolytes (principally sodium), consumption of regular meals, and adequate fluid intake are sufficient, in all but the most exceptional circumstances, to maintain electrolyte homeostasis. Despite the suggestion of large deficits of potassium stores with concomitant muscular weakness in individuals who train exhaustively on repeated days [35], Costill and Miller [16] and Costill [17] present evidence indicating that this not the case, even when dietary potassium intake is extremely low.

The Preevent Meal

The timing and composition of the meal consumed prior to an athletic event or competition have elicited much controversy [4]. This overrated meal has been readily manipulated, often based on unsound nutritional principles, in hopes of attaining a competitive advantage. Although the preevent meal is unlikely to influence performance, at least in short duration events, most authorities recommend the following practices [4,13,16,17,20].

In terms of timing, the object is to ensure that the stomach and upper bowel are empty at the time of the event. As gastrointestinal motility may be reduced by emotional tension, this meal should be consumed three to four hours prior to the event [4,16]. For endurance events, a light carbohydrate meal (500 kilocalories) low in protein and fat is recommended [16]. Protein and fat (as in steak and fried potatoes) are digested slowly and are not utilized readily as fuels during the event [16]. Concentrated sugars (honey, candy, soft drinks) have been promoted for athletes the hour preceding endurance exercise. However, their consumption may result in gastrointestinal distress and impaired performance or earlier exhaustion [4,16]. For long distance runners or persons in training who may become susceptible to dehydration, ingestion of 400 to 600 milliliters of cold water 10 to 15 minutes prior to performance is advisable [14].

During Performance

As thirst is not a sensitive indicator of fluid needs for athletes during training and prolonged periods of competition in warm environments, athletes should force themselves to drink fluids in excess of their perceived needs [4,16]. Even partial rehydration can minimize the risks of overheating and stress on the circulatory system. One investigator has noted that a psychological lift is given to athletes who consume liquids during exercise [36]. To be readily available, ingested fluids must quickly leave the stomach. Thus factors which affect gastric emptying such as the volume, temperature, osmolarity of the replacement fluid are of significance. While large volumes (up to 600 milliliters) of fluid empty rapidly from the stomach, they cause gastric distress for the athlete. Therefore, it is preferable to drink small volumes of fluid more frequently (200 to 300 milliliters every 15 minutes) Cold drinks offer the advantages of emptying more rapidly from the stomach and at the same time enhancing body cooling. Sugars and electrolytes should be used sparingly, if at all, in replacement fluids as they elevate the osmolarity of the drink and impair gastric emptying. In most situations plain water is preferred.

Glycogen Loading

Initial stores of muscle and liver glycogen play a large part in determining success or failure in endurance-type activities lasting 60 minutes or longer (for example, distance running, long duration cycling, cross-country skiing) [4,16,17,27-29,37]. Glycogen loading or muscle glycogen supercompensation is a dietary regimen known to increase muscle glycogen storage well above normal levels. There have been slight modifications, but basically the procedure, initiated about a week prior to competition, involves exercising the athlete to the point of exhaustion during which time muscle glycogen levels are significantly decreased. This also stimulates the muscle's glycogen synthetase activity which facilitates muscle glycogen storage once a high carbohydrate diet is fed. A mixed diet based on the four food groups is fed during these first three days. For the remaining days of the week, a high carbohydrate (75% to 90%) diet is consumed, and exercise/training is drastically reduced to spare glycogen stores. The result, which is localized in the exercising muscles, is about a two-to-threefold increase in muscle glycogen storage compared with that of the unexercised muscle [16]. Application of glycogen loading also benefits performance at high altitudes (8,000 feet) such as mountain climbing where oxygen is less available and greater demands are placed on the anaerobic metabolism of carbohydrate (glycogen storage). The procedure is of no value for short (or intermittent) strenuous events such as football [38].

The type of carbohydrate (simple versus complex) fed during the glycogen loading procedure makes little difference to the rate and quantity of muscle glycogen stored [16]. However, complex carbohydrates (pasta, bread) may be preferred as they produce a longer lasting insulin stimulation and blood glucose elevation. Glycogen storage in an athlete can be monitored by the temporary change in body weight (one to two kilograms) as 2.7 grams of water are stored with each gram of glycogen [4]. The procedure is to be used cautiously and selectively with consideration of possible metabolic and nutritional side-effects [3,4,16,20,39]. Electrocardiographic changes have been shown in at least one participant, and therefore glycogen loading is potentially harmful for the cardiac rehabilitation type runner [3,15].

Weight Gain/Loss

To effectively compete, athletes must attain their appropriate weight, and simultaneously be well nourished, well hydrated, and have a healthy minimum energy reserve as fat [40]. In certain athletic events such as heavyweight wrestling and some positions in football, an increase in body weight may optimize performance. In other sports such as gymnastics or long-distance running a leaner body weight may confer greater efficiency of movement [4,10,41,42]. For the athlete, like the nonathlete who wishes to change his or her body weight, a well-planned and supervised weight control program is emphasized. Weight change should be accomplished gradually (± one to two pounds per week) by moderately adjusting energy balance: energy intake in relation to energy expenditure. Diet modifications for either gaining or losing weight should be based on the four food groups to assure optimal intake of all essential nutrients [6,8,40].

The aim of a weight-gaining program should be to increase lean body mass, that is, muscle, as opposed to body fat. Muscle mass can be increased only by muscle work supported by an appropriate increase in dietary intake, not by any special food, vitamin, drug, or hormone [40].

An estimate of existing and desired body fat should be a prerequisite of the athlete's weight reduction program. In sports such as wrestling, gymnastics, and distance running, about 5% of body weight as fat is considered a healthy minimum. Body fat can be reduced by a modest decrease in food intake and an increase in energy expenditure. One hour of appropriate conditioning can increase energy expenditure by 250 to 750 kilocalories [6,40].

Unfortunately, starvation, semistarvation, and dehydration are all-too-common practices among high school and college wrestlers attempting to abruptly reduce body weight to make a lower weight classification [4,7,10, 43,44]. Such practices will not only impair performance (that is, endurance) but also may endanger health. Dehydration resulting from any means (ketogenic diet, water deprivation, salt deprivation, or diuretics) impairs circulatory function and eventually physical work capacity [4]. Starvation and semistarvation cause weight loss at the expense of lean body tissue rather than fat. This is particularly serious in highly-trained wrestlers who already have a low body fat content. For young competitors, such practices could compromise normal growth [4,40].

Special Concerns

Sports Anemia

This appears to be a transient condition of borderline low hemoglobin levels sometimes observed in athletes during the early stages of a strenuous physical training program [4,20,45]. Theoretically, as total body hemoglobin is related to maximal oxygen uptake, muscular endurance of an individual participating in aerobic type activities could be compromised by low hemoglobin levels. However, its cause and significance are unknown [4]. Various hypotheses have been advanced with respect to its etiology. Perhaps it is a physiological adaptation to training [20]. An increased susceptibility of red blood cells to lysis during exercise which in turn is related to the quality and quantity of dietary protein has been proposed [4,45–47]. And loss of iron in sweat has been presented as an explanation [14]. Whether or not the condition affects physical working capacity is unknown.

Of more serious consideration is the dietary iron intake of women during childbearing years and teenage boys, both of whom have high iron requirements [4,7]. Iron deficiency anemia will adversely affect performance as the oxygen carrying capacity of the blood is reduced. In most cases, iron needs can be met by diet, or by iron supplements for those clinically diagnosed as iron deficient. Unless there is actual measurable iron deficiency, large doses of iron supplements are contraindicated [4].

Food Faddism

A discussion of nutrition and performance would be incomplete without mention of food faddism. Unfortunately, misconceptions and ignorance concerning food selections among athletes are widespread [7,21]. Darden [48] gives two basic reasons for this. First, coaches and athletes are under great pressure to win at all costs; and second, athletes have a tremendous desire to believe in almost anything that will turn them into champions.

Popular among athletes are various ergogenic or work-enhancing dietary aids: glucose and dextrose, honey, gelatin, lecithin, wheat germ oil, yeast powder, phosphates, and vitamins [4]. While it is recognized that any one of the above may confer psychological benefits to the athlete, the vast majority of claims regarding their ergogenic effect is without scientific documentation. Furthermore, their indiscriminate use may impede performance and create unnecessary health problems.

Deficiencies of vitamins can be damaging to work performance due to their role in metabolic pathways. However, this does not mean that vitamin supplementation for athletes who already are well nourished will further improve performance. In particular, vitamin C, vitamin E, and the B-complex vitamins have been studied in this respect. There is a general consensus among investigators that if the athlete consumes a nutritionally balanced diet, vitamin supplements are unnecessary, do not enhance performance, and in the case of fat-soluble vitamins A, D, and E which are stored in the body, may lead to toxic effects [4,17,20,49].

While certain foods and food constituents have been overemphasized on the alleged basis of improving performance, use of other foods has been discouraged [4]. Milk fits into this latter category. Coaches and trainers have restricted athletes' milk consumption during training and before an athletic event on the supposition that milk contributes to cottonmouth (a dryness or discomfort in the mouth due to decreased activity of salivary glands), cuts speed and wind, and causes stomach upset due to curdling in the stomach. Studies show that there is no basis for restricting milk and milk products for the athlete [4]. Cottonmouth appears to be due to emotional stress and fluid loss; performance is not reduced when milk is included in the diet; and milk curdling which is a natural and necessary part of digestion, does not cause stomach upset. More importantly, milk supplies the athlete with valuable nutrients such as calcium, good quality protein, vitamin A, and riboflavin [4].

References

1. U.S. Department of Health, Education, and Welfare. *Healthy People. The Surgeon General's Report On Health Promotion And Disease Prevention.* DHEW (PHS) Publ. No. 79–55071, 1979.

2. Hanley, D.F. *Nutr. Today* 14:22, 1979.

3. National Dairy Council. *Dairy Council Digest* 46:7, 1975.

4. Williams, M.H. *Nutritional Aspects Of Human Physical And Athletic Performance.* Springfield, Illinois: Charles C. Thomas, 1976.

5. Parizkova, J., and Rogozkin, V.A. (Eds.). *Nutrition, Physical Fitness, and Health.* Baltimore, MD.: University Park Press, 1978.

6. Katch, F.I., and McArdle, W.D. *Nutrition, Weight Control, and Exercise.* Boston, Mass.: Houghton Mifflin Co., 1977.

7. Smith, N.J. *Food For Sport.* Palo Alto, Calif.: Bull Publ. Co., 1976.

8. Briggs, G.M., and Calloway, D.H. (Eds.). *Bogert's Nutrition and Physical Fitness* (10th ed.). Philadelphia: W.B. Saunders Co., 1979. Pp. 527–539.

9. Lincoln, A. *Food For Athletes.* Chicago, Illinois: Contemporary Books, Inc., 1979.

10. Smith, N.J. In American Academy of Pediatrics, *Pediatric Nutrition Handbook.* Evanston, Illinois: American Academy of Pediatrics, 1979. Pp. 427–435.

11. Darden, E. *Nutrition and Athletic Performance.* Pasadena, Calif.: The Athletic Press, 1976.

12. Young, D.R. *Physical Performance Fitness and Diet.* Springfield, Illinois: Charles C. Thomas, 1977.

13. Higdon, H. *The Complete Diet Guide for Runners and Other Athletes.* Mountain View, Calif.: World Publ., 1978.

14. Buskirk, E.R. *Postgrad. Med.* 61:229, 1977.

15. The American Dietetic Association. *J. Am. Diet. Assoc.* 76:437, 1980.

16. Costill, D.L. and Miller, J.M. *Int. J. Sports Med.* 1:2, 1980.

17. Costill, D.L. *A Scientific Approach To Distance Running.* Los Altos, Calif.: Tafnews Press, 1979.

18. Hursh, L.M. *Nutr. Today* 14:18, 1979.

19. Cronin, F.J. *Family Economics Rev.* Spring: 10, 1980.

20. Vitousek, S.H. *Nutr. Today* 14:10, 1979.

21. Bentivegna, A., Kelley, E.J., and Kalenak, A. *Phys. Sports Med.* 7:99, 1979.

22. Consolazio, C.F., Johnson, H.L., Nelson, R.A., Dramise, J.G., and Skala, J.H. *Am. J. Clin. Nutr.* 28:29, 1975.

23. Felig, P., and Wahren, J. *N. Engl. J. Med.* 293:1078, 1975.

24. Hanley, D.F. *Nutr. Today* 14:5, 1979.

25. Strauzenberg, S.E., Schneider, F., Donath, R., Zerbes, H., and Kohler, E. *Bibl. Nutr. Dieta.* 27:133, 1979.

26. Koivisto, V., Soman, V., Nadel, E., Tamborlane, W.V., and Felig, P. *Fed. Proc.* 39:1481, 1980.

27. Consolazio, C.F., and Johnson, H.L. *Am. J. Clin. Nutr.* 25:85, 1972.

28. Lewis, S., and Gutin, B. *Am. J. Clin. Nutr.* 26:1011, 1973.

29. Martin, B., Robinson, S., and Robertshaw, D. *Am. J. Clin. Nutr.* 31:62, 1978.

30. Harger, B.S., Miller, J.B., and Thomas, J.C. *JAMA* 228:482, 1974.

31. Consolazio, C.F. In J.I. McKigney and H.N. Munro (Eds.). *Nutrient Requirements in Adolescence.* Cambridge, Mass.: MIT Press, 1976. Pp. 203–221.

32. Claremont, A.D., Costill, D.L., Fink, W., and Van Handel, P. *Med. Sci. Sports.* 8:239, 1976.

33. Consolazio, C.F. In *Symposia of the X International Congress of Nutrition.* Japan: Victory-Sha Press, 1976. Pp. 183–185.

34. American College of Sports Medicine. *Med. Sci. Sports.* 7:7, 1975.

35. Lane, H.W., Roessler, G.S., Nelson, E.W., and Cerda, J.J. *Am. J. Clin. Nutr.* 31:838, 1978.

36. Johnson, D.J. *J. Sports Med.* 15:138, 1975.

37. Bergstrom, J., Hermansen, L., Hultman, E., et al. *Acta. Physiol. Scand.* 71:140, 1967.

38. MacDougall, J.D., Ward, G.R., Sale, D.G., and Sutton, J.R. *J. Appl. Physiol.* 42:129, 1977.

39. Jette, M., Pelletier, O., Parker, L., and Thoden, J. *Am. J. Clin. Nutr.* 31:2140, 1978.

40. Smith, N.J. *JAMA* 236:149, 1976.

41. Freyschuss, U., and Melcher, A. *Scand. J. Clin. Lab. Invest.* 38:753, 1978.

42. Niinimaa, V., Dyon, M., and Shephard, R.J. *Med. Sci. Sports* 10:91, 1978.

43. Sproles, C.B., Smith, D.P., Byrd, R.J., and Allen, T.E. *J. Sports Med.* 16:98, 1976.

44. Vaccaro, P., Zauner, C.W., and Cade, J.R. *J. Sports Med.* 16:45, 1976.

45. Consolazio, C.F., and Takahashi, T. In *Symposia of the X International Congress of Nutrition.* Japan: Victory-Sha Press, 1976. Pp. 174–176.

46. Shiraki, K., Yamada, T., Ashida, T., and Yoshimura, H. In *Symposia of the X International Congress of Nutrition.* Japan: Victory-Sha Press, 1976. Pp. 181–182.

47. Shiraki, K., Yamada, T., and Yoshimura, H. *Japan J. Physiol.* 27:413, 1977.

48. Darden, E.J. *Home Econ.* 69:40, 1977.

49. Lawrence, J.D., Bower, R.C., Richl, W.P., et al. *Am. J. Clin. Nutr.* 28:205, 1975.

8 The Adult Diabetic and Exercise

Lee N. Cunningham, D.P.E.

Introduction

The use of exercise in the treatment of diabetes is not new. Exercise was suggested as a therapy for diabetes in India as early as 600 B.C. The world-renowned diabetologist, Dr. Elliott P. Joslin of Boston, described the treatment of diabetes as a triad consisting of insulin, exercise, and diet. Joslin was an advocate of exercise prior to the discovery of insulin in 1921, and he continued to stress the value of balancing the insulin dose and the dietary intake with exercise even after insulin became available. However, as time passed, less interest in exercise as an integral part of the treatment triad has been observed. The value of exercise in the treatment of diabetes is recognized by most physicians and teaching hospitals as secondary to the delivery of insulin. This approach to treating diabetes is valid since the data supporting exercise as a management mode is minimal. Only one study has been published over the past ten years which has reported the chronic effects of exercise on insulin-dependent diabetics [12]. Several studies have been reported regarding the effects of training on non-insulin-dependent diabetics; however, these results are equivocal [30,37,39]. Excellent review articles relating the effects of acute exercise on diabetic patients have been published [16,44,45]. Despite the lack of scientific documentation regarding exercise training, clinical observations do suggest that properly prescribed endurance exercise can smooth out the management of diabetes which may result in the prevention or delay of diabetic vascular disease.

In prescribing exercise for the diabetic patient, two distinct programs must be established. All diabetics must be evaluated and assigned to an exercise program based upon whether or not they have vascular complications. The diabetic is 25 times more susceptible to blindness, 17 times more susceptible to kidney disease, 5 times more susceptible to gangrene and amputation, and twice as prone to heart disease than the nondiabetic [13]. Those patients who have been screened and who are without vascular complications may be assigned to the regular adult fitness program. Patients with vascular complications (that is, retinopathy, nephropathy, coronary heart disease, or peripheral vascular disease) should be assigned to a cardiac rehabilitation program until they reach the exit criteria for inclusion into the adult fitness phase. The identification of vascular complications must be made by the patient's personal physician, and permission for participation in such a program must be obtained.

Is there a diabetic exercise program? The answer, of course, is no. The exercise prescription is written in the very same manner as for the non-diabetic adult once the initial screening has been completed. This chapter will discuss exercise for the diabetic without vascular complications and offer some suggestions for making a diabetic patient's exposure to an exercise program a pleasant experience based upon the best diabetic research data on acute exercise. Little is known about exercise for diabetic patients with retinopathy, kidney disease, or peripheral vascular disease. Therefore, patients must rely on their personal physicians for advice or await future research findings for guidelines. At present, diabetic patients with heart disease in particular and mild forms of the other diabetic complications are initially assigned to a cardiac rehabilitation program.

Diabetes

Diabetes is a condition characterized by insulin deficiency causing an abnormal fuel-hormone response particularly when challenged by the ingestion of foodstuffs [8,40]. The abnormal fuel-hormone response is characterized by decreased storage and utilization of fuels resulting in elevated levels of glucose, free fatty acids, and ketones. The abnormal fuel-hormone response is probably due to the insulin secretory mechanism of the beta cells of the pancreas, a faulty insulin receptor site on the cell surface of liver, adipose, and muscle tissue, or a metabolic defect within the cell itself. Metabolic abnormalities are considered to be the major cause leading to the development of vascular complications in diabetic patients [7]. Consequently, it is important to control blood glucose as close to normal as possible [8,15]. However, the extent to which glucose is controlled and its relationship to vascular complications are still somewhat controversial [41]. Nevertheless, all groups do agree that some control of blood glucose is important in the therapy regimen.

There are two basic types of diabetes [35]. Persons with diabetes may be classified as being insulin-dependent (IDDM) or non-insulin-dependent (NIDDM). A general summary of these two types of diabetes is shown in table 8-1. The IDDMs are usually under 20 years of age at onset of diabetes; as a group they comprise less than 10% of the diabetic population. Their symptoms of diabetes are acute, metabolic ketoacidosis is frequent, insulin reactions are frequent, insulin production is decreased, the potential for developing maximal performance capacity is reduced, and hyperglycemia is associated with marked reductions in glucose storage and utilization. The NIDDM is generally characterized as being over 40 years of age at onset of

Table 8-1

Summary of the Differences between Insulin-Dependent (IDDM) and Non-Insulin-Dependent (NIDDM) Diabetes

	Insulin-Dependent	*Non-Insulin-Dependent*
Age at onset	Usually under 20	Usually over 40
Proportion of all diabetics	Less than 10%	Greater than 90%
Appearance of symptoms	Acute or subacute	Slow
Metabolic ketoacidosis	Frequent	Rare
Obesity at onset	Uncommon	Common
Beta cells	Decreased	Variable
Insulin	Decreased	Variable
Family history of diabetes	Uncommon	Common

diabetes; over 90% of all diabetics are of this type. In this group, the appearance of symptoms are slow; individuals show a delayed insulin response to a feeding. A family history of diabetes is common, and hyperglycemia is primarily associated with the failure of the liver to retain glucose and a small impairment in glucose oxidation.

Treatment of the Insulin-Dependent Diabetic

The treatment of the insulin-dependent diabetic involves insulin replacement therapy. This must be appropriately balanced with the dietary intake and energy expenditure. The plan of treatment is to normalize the storage and utilization of metabolic fuels by attempting to maintain blood glucose as close to normal as would be feasible. Improved management programs involve the use of various insulins which act at different time periods throughout the day (figure 8-1). In general, most IDDMs will take a combination of quick acting insulin which peaks in two to three hours and an intermediate acting insulin which peaks in seven to eight hours but has a lasting effect over the whole day. Many IDDMs may be taking multiple insulin injections, the most common of which is the split dose. The patient will take about two-thirds of the daily dosage in the morning and the other one-third before supper or at bedtime.

The exercise leader will need to suggest a training schedule which avoids the time periods when the insulin is peaking and to carefully plan a feeding schedule prior to exercise for the patient who might be susceptible to insulin

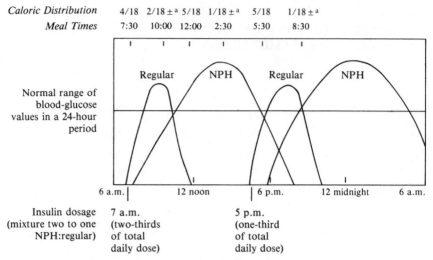

Caloric Distribution   4/18   2/18 ± [a] 5/18   1/18 ± [a]   5/18   1/18 ± [a]

Meal Times   7:30   10:00   12:00   2:30   5:30   8:30

Insulin dosage   7 a.m.   5 p.m.
(mixture two to one   (two-thirds   (one-third
NPH:regular)   of total   of total
daily dose)   daily dose)

[a]The quantity of food consumed as between-meal snacks (and thus the proportion of the daily caloric allotment) is varied with decreased or increased physical activity.

Figure 8–1. A Schematic Illustration of the Relationship of Food and Insulin.

Source: Jackson, R.L., and Guthrie, R.A., *The Child with Diabetes Mellitus,* The Upjohn Company, 1975. Reprinted with permission.

Note: The patient's daily food is given as three meals and three between-meal snacks (which is the most common and desirable pattern of food intake for nondiabetic American children). Insulin is given as two doses daily of a two to one mixture of NPH:regular. Two-thirds of the total daily dose is given in the morning and the remaining one-third is given in late afternoon. Regular insulin takes effect quickly and lasts for only four to six hours. NPH insulin, on the other hand, acts for a longer period and lasts for about 12 to 14 hours. Thus, the regimen provides for maintenance of blood-glucose levels as normal as possible for the diabetic child throughout a 24-hour period, and it helps prevent both urinary spilling of glucose and hypoglycemia.

reactions (low blood glucose levels). In general, to avoid these episodes of exercise-induced hypoglycemia the training program might be conducted within three hours following a meal. In addition to insulin therapy, a carefully planned diet of 50% to 55% carbohydrate, 12% to 20% protein, and the remainder of the calories in fat is suggested for the diabetic by the American Diabetes Association [2]. The diet must adequately supply the energy and nutritional requirements and must be planned in association with the insulin regimen and the exercise plan. The IDDM is not generally overweight or obese; consequently, a diet restricted in calories for weight loss is not required. Nevertheless, it would be important for the exercise leader to have knowledge of both the insulin program and dietary intake and to regularly discuss these components of the treatment regimen with the patient. Knowledgeable IDDMs with an awareness of their diabetes will have a good sense of how exercise fits into the therapy regimen. The newly diagnosed IDDM will be the least knowledgeable about the three factors of treatment. However, in these individuals the diabetes is generally more easily managed since a small amount of insulin is still produced by the pancreas.

Treatment of the Non-Insulin-Dependent Diabetic

Non-insulin-dependent diabetics (NIDDMs) comprise about 90% of the diabetic population. Consequently, they should be the most common type of diabetic encountered in an adult exercise program. Once again, the major deficit is insufficient insulin secretion although hyperinsulinemia may be exhibited in some patients during fasting. However, the smaller change from basal to peak insulin levels in response to feeding is a characteristic of these patients [16]. That is, the insulin response to a carbohydrate meal is delayed, reaching peak values in about two hours. Normal controls exhibit peak insulin in response to carbohydrate ingestion in about one hour. NIDDMs exhibit less liver retention of glucose, which explains the increased blood sugar in the circulation after a meal, and a somewhat lower rate of utilization of glucose by muscle and adipose tissue. A majority of NIDDMs are overweight or obese; therefore, the decreased oxidation rates for carbohydrates may be associated with the interaction of insulin at the cell surface or within the cell itself.

Theoretically, endurance exercise programs may have great potential for the restoration of normal metabolism since both a loss of weight and physical training seem to stimulate the action of insulin. That is, insulin-mediated glucose uptake is enhanced by increasing insulin-binding sensitivity [25,27]. The increased oxidation of metabolic fuel [12,38] and the increased storage of glycogen [32] may serve to normalize metabolism. This may result in improved glucose tolerance following exercise training in NIDDMs [39]. This hypothesis is somewhat controversial since others have failed to obtain similar findings [27,28]. In well-trained nondiabetics and in obese subjects following endurance training, lower levels of insulin were required to dispose of a glucose load [5,26,29,31]. This finding suggests a more efficient use of insulin. Whether or not there is an actual improvement in the rate of glucose storage and utilization is not clear from these studies.

Most insulin-dependents are treated with dietary regimen and/or oral medications. In those patients treated with oral agents, the dosage must be reduced or eliminated when an exercise program is undertaken. These oral agents can produce clinical hypoglycemia under proper conditions. The field of sports science has not fully capitalized on the value of endurance training for these patients. Some studies are currently underway to establish if endurance training in NIDDMs can normalize fuel metabolism.

Benefits of Physical Activity for the Diabetic

Since the primary defect in diabetes is insulin deficiency, any intervention which would increase the efficiency of insulin should be beneficial. Therefore, the beneficial effects of increasing insulin sensitivity and decreasing glucose intolerance would be to smooth out the management of diabetes and to potentially reduce the development of vascular complications. Consequently, the primary effects of endurance training in diabetic patients would occur within the metabolic system. These beneficial changes would include increased insulin sensitivity, the normalization of fuel oxidation rates, increased oxidative enzymes, and increased maximal oxygen consumption. The cardiovascular effects, which are important but probably secondary to the metabolic effects, would include a lowering of hemoglobin A_{Ic} (low levels indicates good control), decreased triglycerides, increased HDL-cholesterol, a reduction of resting blood pressure, improved peripheral circulatory characteristics, increased oxygen transport, and increased cardiac dynamics.

The training effects which result from endurance exercise are shown in table 8–2. Many of these effects have been documented in diabetic patients. Other effects such as increased cardiac dynamics, where the research data is minimal, have been extrapolated from studies performed with nondiabetic subjects. These training effects, when taken together, suggest important implications for the management of diabetes which may lead to the possible prevention or delay of vascular complications.

Table 8–2
Benefits of Regular Endurance Exercise for the Diabetic Patient

Metabolic Effects	Cardiovascular Effects
Increased insulin sensitivity (insulin requirements)	Decreased hemoglobin A_{Ic}
	Decreased triglycerides
Normalization of fuel oxidation rates	Increased HDL-cholesterol
Increased oxidative enzymes	Lower resting blood pressure
Increased storage of glycogen	Improved peripheral circulatory characteristics
Increased amino acid uptake	
Increased maximal oxygen uptake	Increased oxygen transport
	Increased cardiac dynamics

Exercise Metabolism for the Diabetic

All of the acute studies regarding the diabetic's exercising have been undertaken with insulin-dependent (IDDM) subjects. Therefore, the comments made in this section will be related to IDDMs in particular. In some cases, however, it is possible to extrapolate these data to non-insulin-dependents (NIDDMs) during acute exercise.

The IDDMs must be under at least moderate metabolic control if daily exercise is to be of value. In a group of ketotic diabetics (poorly controlled), an increase in blood glucose was noted during 40 to 45 minutes of exercise on a bicycle ergometer [3,46]. However, when the diabetes was under good control, a fall in blood glucose was noted. This reduction in blood glucose is thought to be therapeutically valuable. Consequently, the metabolism must be brought under control with proper insulinization before undertaking the daily exercise session.

Ketosis (poor control) can be identified by the routine testing of urine which is a suggested daily health care procedure for the diabetic. In fact, most diabetologists recommend that diabetic patients keep a log of insulin dosage, urine testing, and dietary information. The exercise leaders may ask the IDDMs to share this data with them and may suggest that the IDDMs record exercise time in the log as well.

Exercise training may play an important role in conjunction with metabolic regulation by any of the new insulin delivery systems. The two systems which are receiving the most research attention at present are the closed-loop artificial beta-cell unit (artificial pancreas) and the open-loop insulin infusion pump. The purpose of these devices is to manage diabetes better. In a recent study a group of conventionally controlled IDDM patients were challenged by a 100 gram glucose drink following an overnight fast and a light exercise bout [17]. The subjects were given their usual insulin dosage 30 minutes prior to the glucose ingestion. The data clearly showed an abnormal hormone-fuel profile over the three hours of the test when compared to normal controls. However, these hormones and fuels were normalized when controlled by an artificial beta-cell unit which monitored blood glucose and infused insulin over a four-day period. The question may be asked, "If insulin infusion can normalize metabolic fuel storage and total body oxidation rates, then why include exercise in the management regimen?" The artificial pancreas is only a tool for short-term metabolic regulation. The end point should not be machine regulation but the retention of normal metabolism long after the patient has left the hospital. Exercise regimens in conjunction with any of the newer management methods (insulin-pumps or multiple injections) would show the greatest potential for retaining metabolic control in IDDMs. The exercise leader will certainly encounter this technology in the immediate future.

Hypoglycemia resulting from low or rapidly falling blood glucose levels is a potential hazard for the exercising IDDM. Subjects who were in the artificial pancreas experiment were exercised for 15 minutes at 40% of their maximal oxygen consumption three hours following the ingestion of 100 grams of glucose [18]. Glucose levels fell from 4 mg/ml to 3.5 mg/ml during the exercise session prior to treatment by the artificial pancreas. Following the four days of treatment, when the glucose was normalized by an insulin infusion, no decrease in blood glucose was noted. Hypoglycemia may be explained by the inhibition of glucose production by the effect of insulin on the liver while the utilization of glucose by muscle increased by 7- to 20-fold. The net effect is rapidly falling glucose levels due to the imbalance between production and utilization. One could predict from these data that with one hour of exercise, when the patient is under conventional therapy, a potentially serious hypoglycemic episode could occur unless some preventive measure is taken.

Recent evidence suggests two possible methods for preventing hypoglycemia in the IDDM during exercise [24,34]. First, a snack of rapidly assimilated carbohydrate such as fruit juice taken 20 to 30 minutes before exercise is suggested. It takes only about 5 to 7 minutes for some of the snack to be metabolized. However, major gains in available fuel is probably not realized until 20 to 30 minutes following the ingestion of the feeding [11]. If the exercise is prolonged over several hours such as hiking, skiing, or canoeing these snacks should be taken every 30 minutes to one hour depending upon the intensity or the type of exercise. Second, when under conventional insulin therapy, the injection site may be important because the pumping effect of the working muscles tends to more rapidly remove insulin from the injection site, thus further exaggerating the hypoglycemia [24,27]. Therefore, it is suggested that an abdominal injection site be used during leg exercise such as running, hiking, or biking. Conversely, when using the arms in an activity such as rowing or canoeing, the thigh would be an appropriate injection site. A smaller drop in blood glucose was observed when this particular experiment was completed in the laboratory [24].

In summary, it seems important not only to use a nonexercising injection site but to take a carbohydrate snack prior to exercise. Zinman reported a significant drop in blood glucose despite administering only 25% of the regular daily insulin dose [47]. Etzwiler has suggested cutting the insulin by 50% while hiking or canoeing for a day or for several days [15]. A backpacking experience with teenage IDDMs showed that even when the daily insulin dosage was cut by 75% most of the hikers showed negative urine tests when they reached camp in the evening. The elimination of insulin completely on very active days is unwise. Berger and coworkers have shown a permissive effect of insulin which is necessary for normal uptake of glucose by muscle, liver, and adipose tissue [4]. Consequently, regular

Table 8–3
Summary of Results from a Survey of Diabetic Runners

Insulin Dose	%	Food Intake	%
No change	61	No change	62
Decreased insulin (2 to 10) units	14	Ate extra food before running	27
Decreased insulin only for race or long run	19	Ate extra food after running	4
Took insulin after running	4	Ate extra food before and after running	4
Took insulin after running (race only)	2	Other	3

Source: Flood, T.M. Who's running. *Diabetes Forecast,* March-April, 1979, p.22. Reprinted with permission. Copyright © 1979 by the American Diabetes Association.

carbohydrate feedings in association with prolonged exercise are necessary. The amount of carbohydrate and the frequency of the feedings depend upon the duration and intensity of the activity.

The Flood survey of diabetic runners indicated that 61% of those completing the survey made no changes in either insulin dose or food intake in preparation for daily runs (table 8–3). Consequently, once the physical activity becomes part of the person's lifestyle, there is little need to adjust for daily exercise. However, the IDDM who is just beginning a program will need a cut in the insulin requirements, particularly during the first two to three weeks of training. Some runners in this survey reported a drop of 17 units of insulin during the training process.

Cardiovascular Dynamics and the Diabetic

The type of screening the diabetic should undergo prior to initiating an endurance exercise-training program will depend upon the age of the patient, the duration of diabetes, the type of diabetes, associated cardiovascular risk factors, and the extent of any vascular complications. Karlfors administered exercise tests to male diabetics aged 17 to 44 and found that ST-segment changes were correlated to the duration of diabetes and to the degree of retinopathy [23]. Levitas and Dristal tested 40 insulin-dependent (IDDM) patients in the 20- to 30-year-old age group and 14 in the group aged 30 to 40. They found eight patients with a positive stress test, seven of whom had had diabetes for more than 12 years [30]. Leon and colleagues recently reported that significant depressions of the ST-segment occurred in 8% of the 38 non-insulin-dependents (mean age of 57 years, duration of diabetes 4 years) who were stress tested and that another 10% exhibited borderline changes [28]. In a recent study of 60 IDDMs, aged 18 to 30 years

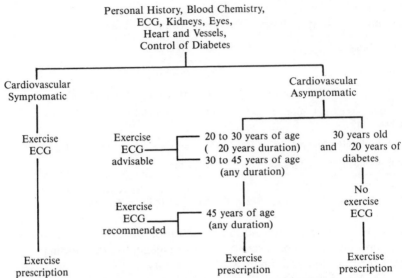

Figure 8-2. Resting Evaluation of Patients for Entry into an Endurance Fitness Program

with a mean duration of diabetes of 10 years, no significant ST-segment depressions or rhythmic changes at any workload up to 90% of the age-adjusted maximal heart rate or during the recovery period was found. These studies seem to indicate that not all diabetics require exercise stress testing. The need for such testing appears to be related to age and duration of diabetes.

A proposed model for making decisions about exercise stress testing for the diabetic adult is shown in figure 8-2. The symptomatic patient must be tested regardless of age or duration of diabetes. In view of the findings for asymptomatic patients under 30 years of age and with less than 20 years of diabetes, a stress test would seem unnecessary, and the exercise prescription can be written. An exercise ECG is advisable for patients aged 20 to 35 years with over 20 years of diabetes, and from 30 to 45 years with over 10 years of diabetes. All diabetics over 45 years of age regardless of duration of diabetes should be exercise stress tested. This proposed model is only a suggestion. The cardiologist or diabetologist must evaluate each patient and then make decisions based upon the medical history. Diabetes has been referred to as accelerated aging. Therefore, the chronological age may not accurately estimate the biological age of the diabetic. The duration of diabetes must also be considered.

The use of heart rate to estimate exercise intensity may be invalid when used with diabetic patients. Several studies have shown that during exercise the heart rate of diabetic subjects was 15 to 30 beats per minute higher at the same percentage of the maximal oxygen consumption when compared to nondiabetic subjects [19,34,46]. It has been suggested that this is related to the extraordinary rise in catecholamines which has been noted in diabetic patients both at rest and during exercise [10]. The overestimation of heart rate would reduce the exercise intensity. This would result in safer exercise particularly for the low-fit, poorly controlled diabetic. As the fitness capacity increases and the diabetes becomes better managed, the span between the catecholamine-induced elevated heart rate and a normal heart rate response is narrowed. On the other hand, patients with cardiac neuropathy will exhibit the opposite heart-rate response. That is, at a similar percentage of the maximal oxygen consumption the diabetic with cardiac neuropathy will exhibit a lower heart rate [21]. Cardiac neuropathy can be identified by the lack of beat-to-beat variation in the cardiac cycle. Consequently, this abnormality should be ruled out during the initial screening by monitoring the resting ECG according to a simple test for autonomic neuropathy devised by Hilsted and Jensen [22].

Most studies comparing maximal oxygen uptake between diabetic and nondiabetic subjects reported no significant differences between groups [12,20,38,46]. These findings may be due to careful subject selection since recent reviews have suggested that IDDM patients without clinically detectable signs of vascular disease and who are nonketotic may exhibit a reduced potential for achieving maximal oxygen consumption [14,33]. This conclusion is based primarily upon hematological and circulatory data which showed that IDDMs have reduced tissue oxygen delivery due to elevated hemoglobin A_{Ic} levels, decreased 2,3 diphosphoglycerate production, increased blood viscosity, decreased plasma volume, and decreased numbers of capillaries per cross-sectional area of muscle tissue.

Peripheral circulation in IDDM subjects was studied recently at the Joslin Research Laboratory. Although the resting minute flow was not significantly different, the diabetic subjects showed significantly greater vasodilation of the peripheral circulation. After three minutes of isometric exercise, the IDDM group exhibited significantly less minute flow and greater vasodilated flow pattern. In addition, IDDMs with duration of diabetes of 15 years showed significantly less arterial elasticity. When these findings were related to levels of endurance fitness, those diabetic patients with high fitness levels showed greater peripheral blood flow and vessel elasticity along the arterial system for any given duration of diabetes. These findings suggest that programs of endurance exercise may delay the time at which severe peripheral circulatory abnormalities may occur.

**A Suggested Program and Some Additional Hints for
Diabetic Patients**

As previously mentioned there are no special exercises for the diabetic. Exercise prescriptions can be written by adapting the best of the available information regarding fitness programming. Tables 8-4, 8-5, and 8-6 illustrate a suggested program which is distributed to patients who attend an optional lecture given weekly at the Joslin Diabetes Center, Inc., Boston. The plan is essentially adopted from the American College of Sports Medicine's position statement for prescribing exercise in healthy adults [1]. Any of the activities shown in table 8-6 may be adopted as the mode of exercise with a great emphasis upon walking. First, walking is a very efficient activity that requires little cost or equipment. Second, walking is basically a safe activity in terms of intensity since the majority of the patients seen in the Diabetes Treatment Unit in Boston are over 50 years of age and have been inactive for many years. Table 8-4 suggests the number of sessions per week, the duration of each activity session, and the total minutes of exercise per week. The prescription is based on time of exercise rather than METS, kilocalories per minute, or aerobic points. Patients may shift into a higher fitness level when they comfortably achieve the required total time per week for that fitness category. This insures progression in the program. The moderate fitness level is a realistic goal for most diabetic patients without vascular disease. The program requires about three hours of endurance exercise at the appropriate intensity per week. The intensity of exercise is determined by a given fitness level and is increased as the person's endurance capacity is increased. Table 8-5 shows the minute heart rates for a given percentage of maximum according to age. Recall that insulin-dependents (IDDMs) will exhibit an elevated minute heart rate during exercise; consequently, they will be working at a reduced percentage of the maximal oxygen consumption. It may take the diabetic a little longer to reach certain training goals, but there is, thus, a built-in safety device to prevent overexertion.

A reduction in the insulin requirements will be noted at the start of the training program for the IDDM. It will take between one to three weeks for the insulin to reach its new level. During that period of time the patient may experience some glucose-insulin fluctuations possibly leading to some episodes of hypoglycemia. The exercise leader will need to have some simple carbohydrate available such as lifesavers, honey, gingerale, sugar cubes, or fruit juice to treat these reactions to insulin. A note of caution is that the diabetic should never leave the exercise center for a jog around town without carrying some simple sugar. Also, it is unwise for the diabetic to run alone. Finally, the need to reduce the daily insulin dosage is a signal that some desirable metabolic changes are occurring. Because so many IDDMs

Table 8–4
Exercise Prescription According to Fitness Level

Fitness Level	Frequency (Sessions/Week)	Duration (Minutes/Session)	Time/Week (Minutes)	Intensity (% Maximal Heart Rate[a])	Type of Activity
Very low	4–6	10–20	40–80	60	—[b]
Low	4–6	15–30	90–120	60–70	—[b]
Moderate	3–5	20–45	90–130	70–80	—[b]
High	3–5	30–60	180–300	70–90	—[b]
Superior (athlete)	5–7	60–120	300–840	80–90	—[b]

Note: Exercise time should only include those periods when the body is in motion. Do not count break time.

[a]See table 8–5.
[b]See table 8–6.

Table 8–5
Exercise Heart Rate by Age

Age	Predicted Maximal Heart Rate	90% Maximum	85% Maximum	80% Maximum	75% Maximum	70% Maximum	65% Maximum	60% Maximum
15	193	174	164	154	145	135	125	116
20	191	172	162	153	143	134	124	115
25	189	170	161	151	142	133	123	113
30	186	167	158	149	140	130	121	111
35	184	166	156	147	138	129	120	110
40	182	164	155	146	137	127	118	109
45	180	162	153	144	135	126	117	108
50	178	160	151	142	134	125	116	107
55	175	158	149	140	131	123	114	105
60	173	156	147	138	130	121	112	104
65	171	154	145	137	128	120	111	103

Note: Monitor the exercise intensity of the exercise session. The percentage of exercise heart rate is found by extending the row of the fitness level (table 8–4) A person in the very low fitness category would plan to train at an intensity which is 60 percent of the maximum age-adjusted heart rate.

Table 8-6

Physical Activities Which Can Be Used to Stimulate a Beneficial Effect in Diabetic Patients

Individual Activities	Team Sports
Walking	Soccer
Running-jogging	Basketball
Bicycling (or stationary)	Volleyball
Swimming	Hockey (ice and field)
Dancing	Lacrosse
Rope skipping	
Skiing (downhill and cross-country)	
Rowing	
Skating	
Badminton	
Golf	
Wrestling	
Fencing	
Stair climbing	
Calisthenics	
Tennis	
Handball	
Squash	
Racquetball	

Note: Any of the physical activities listed above can be used in an exercise program which will be beneficial to the diabetic. These activities have been selected because they place a high energy demand upon the body. How hard these activities are played should be regulated by the appropriate percentage of the maximal heart rate for a given fitness level. The heart rate should be monitored periodically.

are overinsulinized due to a sedentary lifestyle, these adjustments should be expected and are a normal part of the treatment routine.

The diabetic may not need to exercise every day. Some metabolic evidence from obese subjects have shown that a single bout of exercise will decrease the insulin requirement for at least one day. If these data can be extrapolated to both the IDDM and the NIDDM, then the American College of Sports Medicine's suggestion of three to five exercise sessions per week is valid for the diabetic. This response may differ from patient to patient, however. Some diabetics may prefer to exercise daily.

Infection may be a problem for some diabetics. Although the frequency of infections are not increased when compared to the nondiabetic, infections do tend to be more serious. In addition, the healing time for cuts and bruises may be lengthened. This suggests that when the diabetic does come down with a cold or the flu it must not be regarded lightly. The exercise leader must encourage a day or two off to treat the infection and to regulate the diabetes which may be significantly disturbed. Recall that when an out-of-control diabetic (ketotic) exercises, the condition worsens.

Immediate treatment of cuts, blisters, and floor burns is critical if infection is to be curtailed and the healing process facilitated. In addition, the diabetic should invest in proper exercise equipment, particularly footwear. An injury as simple as a blister on the small toe may prevent the diabetic from doing the needed exercise for much longer than might be expected. Therefore, it is important to suggest that any of the high quality running shoes be purchased prior to starting a jogging or even a walking program. This is also important for other sports as well; high quality and comfortable golf shoes, basketball sneakers, racquetball footwear, and so forth, must be selected for the activity.

The adherence to a program, although discussed elsewhere in this book, needs to be mentioned here. Sachs pointed out in chapter 3 that persons who are more prone to the development of disease will be more likely to adhere to an exercise program. Furthermore, many diabetics are extremely goal oriented and desire to prove that diabetes is not a disabling condition. This type of person will adhere to the program. On the other hand, some persons with diabetes may need to be continually encouraged. These persons will use diabetes as the excuse for not continuing participation. The exercise leader must know the personalities of the diabetics in the program and continually encourage them in a positive manner. Unfortunately, the diabetic who needs an exercise program the most will often be the first to drop out.

Summary

Because the diabetic is more prone to vascular complications, a careful screening procedure prior to the exercise program is critical. The organization of exercise training for the adult diabetic should include two distinct programs: first, the adult fitness program for the diabetic without vascular complications, and, second, a cardiac rehabilitation program for diabetics with vascular complications. For the insulin-dependent diabetic, the time of day, the injection site used, the feeding schedule, and the state of metabolic control (nonketotic) are important considerations prior to and during exercise. An endurance training program may be an important adjunct to the therapy regimen for the non-insulin-dependent diabetic since only a small modification of the metabolism is required for normalization. Several disturbances of the cardiovascular system are noted with diabetes such as an elevated heart rate, decreased oxygen transport, reduced peripheral blood flow, and a reduced potential for achieving maximal oxygen consumption. The exercise program for the healthy diabetic is planned in the same manner as for any healthy adult. When taken together, the benefits of regular endurance exercise would seem to be cost effective in terms of fewer sick days and less long-term vascular complications.

References

1. American College of Sports Medicine. The recommended quantity and quality of exercise for developing and maintaining fitness in healthy adults. Position statement. *Med. Sci. Sports* 10:vii-x, 1978.

2. American Diabetic Association. Principles of nutrition and dietary recommendations for individuals with diabetes mellitus: 1979. *Diabetes* 28:1027-1030, 1979.

3. Berger, M., Berchtold, P., Cuppers, H.J., et al. Metabolic and hormonal effects of muscular exercise in juvenile-type diabetics. *Diabetologia* 13:355-365, 1977.

4. Berger, M., Hagg, S., and Ruderman, N.B. Glucose metabolism in perfused skeletal muscle: Interaction of insulin and exercise on glucose uptake. *Biochem. J.* 146:231-238, 1975.

5. Bjorntorp, P., DeJounge, C., Sjostrom, L., and Sullivan, L. The effect of physical training on insulin production in obesity. *Metabolism* 8:631-637, 1970.

6. Bjorntorp, P., Fahlen, M., Grimby, G., et al. Carbohydrate and lipid metabolism in middle-aged, physically well-trained men. *Metabolism* 21:1037-1044, 1972.

7. Brownlee, M., and Cahill, G.F., Jr. Diabetic control and vascular complications. In R. Paoletti and A.M. Gotto, Jr. (Eds.), *Atherosclerosis Reviews*. Vol. 4. New York: Raven Press, 1979. Pp. 29-70.

8. Cahill, G.F., Jr. Physiology of insulin. *Diabetes* 20:785-799, 1971.

9. Cahill, G.F., Jr., Etzwiler, D.D., and Freinkel, N. Control and diabetes. *N. Engl. J. Med.* 294:1004-1005, 1976.

10. Christensen, M.J., Galbo, H., Hansen, J.F., Hesse, B., Richter, E., and Trap-Jensen, J. Catecholamines and exercise. *Diabetes* 28 (suppl. 1): 58-62, 1979.

11. Costill, D.L., Bennett, A., Branam, G., and Eddy, D. Glucose ingestion at rest and during prolonged exercise. *J. Appl. Physiol.* 34:764-769, 1973.

12. Costill, D.L., Cleary, P., Fink, W.J., Foster, C., Ivy, J.L., and Witzman, F. Training adaptations in skeletal muscle of juvenile diabetics. *Diabetes* 28:818-822, 1979.

13. Crofford, O. *Report of the National Commission on Diabetes.* DHEW pub. no. (NIH) 76-1018. Washington, D.C.: Government Printing Office, 1975.

14. Ditzel, J. Oxygen transport impairment in diabetes. *Diabetes* 25 (suppl. 2):832–838, 1976.

15. Etzwiler, D.D. When the diabetic wants to be an athlete. *Phys. Sports Med.* 2:45–50, 1974.

16. Felig, P., Wahren, J., and Hendler, R. Influence of maturity-onset diabetes on splanchnic glucose balance after oral glucose ingestion. *Diabetes* 27:121–126, 1978.

17. Foss, M.C., Vlachokosta, F.V., Cunningham, L.N., and Aoki, T.T. Normalization of hormone-fuel metabolism in insulin dependent diabetic subjects. (Abstract) *Clinical Research* 28:647A, 1980.

18. Foss, M.C., Vlachokosta, F.V., Cunningham, L.N., and Aoki, T.T. Hormone-fuel metabolism during exercise of insulin-dependent diabetic subjects treated with a glucose controlled insulin infusion system. (Abstract) *Clinical Research* 28:647A, 1980.

19. Gundersen, H.J.G. Peripheral blood flow and metabolic control in juvenile diabetes. *Diabetologia* 10:225–231, 1974.

20. Hagen, R.D., Marks, J.F., and Warren, P.A. Physiological responses of juvenile onset diabetic boys to muscular work. *Diabetes* 28:1114–1119, 1979.

21. Hilsted, J., Galbo, H., and Christensen, N.J. Impaired cardiovascular responses to graded exercise in diabetic autonomic neuropathy. *Diabetes* 28:313–319, 1979.

22. Hilsted, J., and Jensen, S.B. A simple test for autonomic neuropathy in juvenile diabetics. *Acta. Med. Scand.* 205:385–387, 1979.

23. Karlfors, T. Haemodynamic studies in male diabetics. *Acta Med. Scand.* 180:45–80, 1966.

24. Koivisto, V.A., and Felig, P. Effects of leg exercise on insulin absorption in diabetic patients. *N. Engl. J. Med.* 298:79–83, 1978.

25. Koivisto, V.A., Soman, V., Conrad, P., Hendler, R., Nadel, E., and Felig, P. Insulin binding to monocytes in trained athletes: changes in the resting state and after exercise. *J. Clin. Invest.* 64:1011–1015, 1979.

26. Krotiewski, M., Mandrukos, K., Sjostrom, K., et al. Effects of long-term physical training on body fat, metabolism and blood pressure in obesity. *Metabolism* 28:650–658, 1979.

27. LeBlanc, J., Nadeau, A., Boulay, M., and Rousseau-Migneron, S. Effects of physical training and adiposity on glucose metabolism and 125I-insulin binding. *J. Appl. Physiol.* 46:235–239, 1979.

28. Leon, A.S., Conrad, J.C., Casal, D.C., and Goetz, F.C. Failure of exercise alone to control maturity-onset diabetes. (Abstract) *Med. Sci. Sports* 12:104, 1980.

29. Leon, A.S., Conrad, J., Hunninghake, D.B., and Serfass, R. Effects of a vigorous walking program on body composition and carbohydrate and lipid metabolism on obese young men. *Am. J. Clin. Nutr.* 33:1776–1787, 1979.

30. Levitas, I.M., and Dristal, J.J. Stress exercise testing of the young diabetic for the detection of unknown coronary artery disease. *Israel J. Med.* 8:345–347, 1972.

31. Lohmann, D., Liebold, F., Heilmann, W., Senger, H., and Pohl, A. Diminished insulin response in highly trained athletes. *Metabolism* 27:521–524, 1978.

32. Maehlum, S., Hostmark, A.T., and Hermansen, L. Synthesis of muscle glycogen during recovery after prolonged severe exercise in diabetic subjects: Effect of insulin deprivation. *Scand. J. Clin. Lab. Invest.* 38:35–39, 1978.

33. McMillan, D.E. Exercise and diabetic microangiopathy. *Diabetes* 28(suppl. 1):103–106, 1979.

34. Murray, T.T., Zinman, B., McClean, P.A., et al. The metabolic response to moderate exercise in diabetic men receiving intravenous and subcutaneous insulin. *J. Clin. Endocrinol. Metab.* 44:708–720, 1977.

35. National Diabetes Group. Classification and diagnosis of diabetes mellitus and other categories of glucose intolerance. *Diabetes* 28:1039–1057, 1979.

36. Proceedings of a Conference on Diabetes and Exercise. *Diabetes* 28(suppl. 1):1–113, 1979.

37. Ruderman, N.B., Ganda, O.P., and Johansen, K. The effect of physical training on glucose tolerance and plasma lipids in maturity-onset diabetes. *Diabetes* 28(suppl. 1):89–92, 1979.

38. Saltin, B., Houston, M., Nygaard, E., Graham, T., and Wahren, J. Muscle fiber characteristics in healthy men and patients with juvenile diabetes. *Diabetes* 28(suppl. 1):93–99, 1979.

39. Saltin, B., Lindgarde, F., Houston, M., Nygaard, E., and Gad, P. Physical training and glucose tolerance in middle-aged men with chemical diabetes. *Diabetes* 28(suppl. 1):30–32, 1979.

40. Sherwin, R., and Felig, P. Pathophysiology of diabetes mellitus. *Med. Clin. N. Amer.* 62, (no. 4):695–711, 1978.

41. Siperstein, M.D., Foster, D.W., Knowles, H.C., Jr., Levine, R., Madison, L.L.,and Roth, J. Control of blood glucose and diabetic vascular disease. *N. Engl. J. Med.* 18:1060–1063, 1977.

42. Standl, E., Lotz, N., Dexel, T.H., Janka, H.U., and Kolb, J.J. Muscle triglyceride in diabetic subjects. *Diabetologia* 18:463–469, 1980.

43. Vignati, L., and Cunningham, L.N. Exercise. In A. Marble (Ed.), *Joslin's Diabetes Mellitus* (12th ed.). Philadelphia: Lea and Febiger. In press.

44. Vranic, M., and Berger, M. Exercise and diabetes mellitus. *Diabetes* 28:147–167, 1979.

45. Wahren, J., Felig, P. and Hagenfeldt, L. Physical exercise and fuel homeostasis in diabetes mellitus. *Diabetologia* 14:213–222, 1978.

46. Wahren, J., Hagenfeldt, L., and Felig, P. Splanchnic and leg

exchange of glucose, amino acids and FFA during exercise in diabetes mellitus. *J. Clin. Invest.* 55:1303–1314, 1975.

47. Zinman, B., Murray, F.T., Vranic, M., et al. Glucoregulation during moderate exercise in insulin treated diabetes. *J. Clin. Endocrinol. Metab.* 45:641–652, 1977.

IV Exercise in Cardiac Rehabilitation

9 Inpatient Cardiac Rehabilitation

Gail Handysides, R.N., M.S.N.

Cardiac rehabilitation means different things to different people, depending on their professional biases. It can mean teaching people about their disease process, physical conditioning, or merely aiding people in adjusting to and coping with a cardiac diagnosis. Cardiac rehabilitation can be a holistic service which facilitates patients in achieving their most desired and realistic physical, psychological, vocational, and even spiritual potentials.

Cardiac rehabilitation has formally been available (with a major focus on physical conditioning) in various centers across the United States for about 30 years. In 1948, Newman advocated supervised walking three to five minutes twice a day during the fourth week of recovery for post-myocardial infarction patients [3]. Ten years later, Torkelson advocated exercise tolerance testing for patients in their seventh post-myocardial infarction week, provided they had ambulated during their fifth and sixth weeks [4]. In 1964, Montefiore Hospital in New York City began a progressive multidisciplinary program for cardiac patients, advocating chair for the second week post-myocardial infarction patients, and monitored ambulation during their third week. In 1967, Dr. Wenger in Atlanta began what is now a widely known program in inpatient cardiac rehabilitation monitoring patients' progressive ambulation and other activities using a 14-step protocol [5]. Research carried out in Scotland and Europe by Groden and Hakkila showed that patients mobilized earlier showed no more complications of heart attack than those mobilized later [1,2]. Numerous studies in the last ten years have continued to document the benefits of education, exercise, and functional activities for patients with a cardiac diagnosis.

The overall benefits of rehabilitation for cardiac inpatients include:

1. Prevention of thromboembolism
2. Prevention of general deconditioning
3. Promotion of psychologic well-being
4. Provision of spiritual comfort
5. Decrease in length of hospital stay
6. An increased awareness of cardiac disease information and modes available for life-style alteration.

At New England Memorial Hospital, the primary program focus is twofold: first, to help patients feel better about themselves physically and emotionally; second, to achieve an optimal level of physical conditioning, functional capacity, and intellectual understanding about heart disease. This is best achieved through a multidisciplinary approach involving the following services:

1. *Physican*—takes a health history and performs a thorough exam. Monitors patient's progress throughout the cardiac rehabilitation course. Performs stress tests and develops target heart rates for patients.
2. *Nurse*—evaluates patients' perceptions of their health histories, takes risk factor histories, and records patients' goals. Performs brief physical assessment and monitors patients with ECG during exercise session. Coordinates team goals and patient education.
3. *Dietician*—takes diet history. Prescribes and instructs patient's diet. Demonstrates alternative methods of cooking and diet planning.
4. *Physical Therapist*—performs physical therapy evaluation. Leads group and individual exercise sessions. Prescribes home exercise and maintenance programs. Instructs patients in exercise rationale, motivation, and so forth.
5. *Occupational Therapist*—performs occupational therapy with a focus on functional activities and goals. Leads group and individual functional activities. Performs counseling on life goals, vocational adjustments, and life stressors.
6. *Chaplain or Social Worker*—evaluates patients for coping mechanisms surrounding illness and readjustments due to heart disease. Provides individual and family counseling.
7. *Others*—perform individual and group instruction. Aid in patient's coping mechanisms and provide individual and family support. Act as resource persons and provide referrals for cardiac rehabilitation.

The others in number seven represent all those who take time to listen to patients, giving them a little of what they want and a lot of what they need. They are available to family members and actively participate in the health promotion process. They practice what they preach, instructing primarily by example. They are the staff nurses, clinical specialists, therapists, health educators, and social workers who take an interest in helping to meet a wide variety of patients' physical, emotional, and spiritual needs. Some of what health professionals do overlaps at times, but this serves to reinforce and motivate compliance, which is the salient payoff for the patients and the professionals in cardiac rehabilitation.

Patients are referred within one to two days of their hospital admission (nonmyocardial infarction diagnoses primarily angina related) or within three to five days postinfarction. All patients are introduced to the scope of

Table 9–1
Standards Checklist For Cardiac Rehabilitation Inpatients

	Date and Initials	Patient Initials
Orientation to cardiac rehabilitation		
Initial interviews and evaluations		
Basic cardiac anatomy and physiology		
Area and size of infarct, collateral circulation		
Pulse taking		
Principles of exercise		
Daily exercise session		
Stress management [a]		
Relaxation [a]		
Vocational guidance [a]		
Energy conservation		
Dietary counseling		
Medication teaching		
Good Life for Your Heart class		
Explanation of cardiac rehabilitation to family		
Home program		
Post-test		

Note: This checklist should be supplemented by documentation in nursing, rehabilitation, or dietary progress notes. In addition to this checklist, cardiac rehabilitation patients should be weighed every Wednesday and charted on the graph if daily weights are not ordered.
[a] If appropriate.

cardiac rehabilitation services available and given the opportunity to refuse the program or refuse services they do not want. Table 9–1 shows the standard checklist which is placed in the chart to document services rendered. A five-step ambulation protocol is placed in the chart by which patients are progressed at their personal physician's discretion. The patient is seen several times a day for physical therapy (15 to 20 minutes in the a.m.) and occupational therapy (15 to 30 minutes in the p.m.), and they may attend heart classes (1:30 to 2:30 p.m. Monday through Friday). They may be seen at other times during the day by the social worker, chaplain, or other health professionals for teaching, depending on their learning readiness which is assessed by the team nurse.

Topics covered in the Good Life for Your Heart class include:

Monday—risk factors, atherosclerosis

Tuesday—cholesterol and triglycerides

Wednesday—exercise, activity, stress management

Thursday—hypertension

Friday—chemicals that affect the heart

Other events which may occur during a patient's stay prior to discharge might include a visit from a cardiac rehabilitation outpatient or for a few patients, a submaximal stress test. Generally, the patients' objectives prior to discharge include: general education, psychologic preparation for discharge, the ability to walk without assistance for a prescribed distance including the ascent and descent of 14 stairs, and receiving appropriate activity guidelines based on their MET level capacity. The staff tries to maintain a flexible approach to patients in terms of both what the patients will be able to do and absorb and what can be expected of the staff in helping them. All of the New England Memorial Hospital Cardiac Rehabilitation staff are trained in basic life support, several have graduate degrees, and all have a zeal for working with people and practicing what they preach—a key factor in program success.

When patients first arrive in the coronary care unit, their initial fear is, "Am I going to make it?" After their conditions have stabilized, they begin to wonder, "Now what do I do with my life? Is this the way I'm going to be for the next 20 years, or will I come back to a normal life?"

Much of the fear of having heart disease can be alleviated through education and time. One of the major goals of cardiac rehabilitation is to educate patients about their risk factors and heart disease. Cardiac rehabilitation offers modes in which patients can alter, modify, or control their life styles to prevent the physical and emotional complications of heart disease. Education begins in the inpatient phase with the Good Life for Your Heart class, a five-day series of lectures on heart-related topics and one-to-one sessions with health professionals on such topics as pulse-taking, medications, stress management, and the benefits of exercise. Wherever possible, family members are encouraged to be present at teaching sessions, not only to aid in the patient's compliance with prescribed treatments but also for their own benefit. In fact, outpatient family members are formally included in learning cardiopulmonary resuscitation, participating in a support-group session, or attending a cooking demonstration.

Each health professional involved in cardiac rehabilitation has unique services to offer the patients. Dieticians take a complete diet history from all cardiac rehabilitation patients and then advise them on their prescribed diets. Patients with an obesity problem are closely monitored with weekly weights, and dietary changes are advised as needed. All patients are encouraged to align their diets with the U.S. dietary goals to lower their fat, cholesterol, and simple sugar intake and to increase their dietary intake of fiber foods such as whole wheat grains, fresh fruits, and vegetables.

Occupational therapists focus on patients' life stressors, life goals, and functional needs. Activity guidelines are given to patients at hospital discharge according to their MET-level capacity and are updated on an outpatient basis. Outpatients who are inactive are assisted by occupational therapists in finding employment or volunteer work or in returning to work if they so desire. Occupational therapists also advise patients on time and stress management and lead relaxation sessions.

Physical therapists lead group and individual exercise sessions and devise home exercise programs and maintenance plans for patients. The program demonstrates that it is just a matter of now building back up to where the person was without going overboard. Patients who express needs in the spiritual or emotional realm are referred to the chaplain or social worker who works with the cardiac rehabilitation program.

All patients undergoing cardiac rehabilitation are discussed at weekly team meetings so that the plan of care for each patient is tailor-made for that individual. Periodic patient evaluations and progress notes are sent to patients' personal physicans including information from each discipline involved. The cardiac rehabilitation physician advises team members on outpatients who have been examined prior to their entrance into the more vigorous 12-week phase of cardiac rehabilitation. This physician also determines patients' exercise target heart rates during the 12-week exercise session. Patients may enter cardiac rehabilitation at any phase with the following three entry levels available: first, the inpatient under the direction of the patient's personal physician; second, the convalescent phase at discharge which includes two exercise sessions a week; and, third, the 12-week phase in which patients are exercised at target heart rate three times per week. Prior to entering the 12-week phase, the cardiac rehabilitation physician supervises the patients' conventional stress test or stress thallium test in determining target heart rates and ascertaining any previously undetected problem areas in the myocardium.

During all exercise sessions, patients are monitored for arrhythmias, and preexercise and postexercise blood pressure readings are taken by the cardiac nurse. The patients' physicians are notified immediately if problems are noted. Exercise sessions consist of warm-up calisthenics, walking or jogging, bike ergometry, and upper-extremity conditioning.

The major goal of cardiac rehabilitation is to return patients to full and productive lives as soon as possible. Cardiac rehabilitation can be considered for any heart patient whether the problem is angina, myocardial infarction, open heart surgery, or merely a high-risk profile. It offers a viable adjunct to conventional treatments such as medication and surgery. It is up to physicians to make the choices that they feel will help their cardiac patients enjoy life to the fullest.

References

1. Groden, B.M. The management of myocardial infarction. *Cardiac Rehabil.* 1:13–16, 1971.

2. Hakkila, J. Finds working ability works. *Chron. Dis. Management* 6:1–10, Jan. 1972.

3. Newman, L.B., Wasserman, R.R., and Borden, C. Productive lining for those with heart disease: the role of phys. medicine and rehabilitation. *Arch. Phys. Med. Rehabil.* 37:137–149, 1956.

4. Torkelson, Leif O. Rehabilitation of the patient with acute myocardial infarction. *J. Chronic Dis.* 17:685–704, 1964.

5. Wenger, N.K., Gilbert, C.A. and Skorpa, M.Z. Cardiac conditioning after myocardial infarction. *Cardiac Rehabil.* 2:17–22, 1971.

10 Outpatient Cardiac Rehabilitation

Nancy V. Dolan, R.N., M.S.N.
and
Christopher T. Coughlin, M.S.

Introduction

The New England Heart Center is a comprehensive, multidisciplinary facility devoted to prevention, detection, rehabilitation, and education. The rehabilitation program is a phase 2 outpatient program.

The center began a little over two years ago, and it was started because of patients' needs. Although cardiac patients were receiving excellent care in hospital settings, it was obvious that this care was required beyond discharge from the hospital. In hospital settings, cardiac patients were afforded the expertise of numerous disciplines. Once discharged, however, they were relegated to the care of the physician where the main focus was medical care. Patients were often left to their own devices to continue with the rehabilitation process. Shorter hospital stays, the physiologic and psychologic consequences of a cardiac event, the life-style changes that were usually recommended, and increased responsibility of patients for their own care, all pointed to a need for more than the acute care setting or average visit to the cardiologist's office.

Description of Facility

The center is not attached to a hospital but is in a large medical office building. The exercising area is light and cheerful with trees outside and plants inside. The staff does not wear uniforms or lab coats, thus downplaying a sick or disease atmosphere. There are facilities to exercise nine patients simultaneously. Equipment includes a treadmill, an arm and bicycle ergometer, a rowing machine, and a small carpeted track. There are facilities to monitor four patients on telemetry and a fully equipped emergency cart with defibrillator. The staff is certified in cardiopulmonary resuscitation, and a cardiologist is always on the premises during exercise sessions.

The atmosphere is consciously light and cheerful to facilitate patient motivation to continue in the program. The nurse, exercise physiologist, and dietitian are present during all sessions so that spontaneous one-to-one counseling does occur.

Patient Population

Patients include people with a prior history of myocardial infarction, coronary artery bypass surgery, and stable angina. Program participation is encouraged as soon as it is medically possible after hospital discharge since this seems to be the most acute period during which these patients require help. Six weeks after a myocardial infarction and about four weeks following coronary artery bypass grafting is the earliest that patients have been seen. In the past two years, there have been 113 patients in the rehabilitation program:

Sex: males = 79% (90)
    females = 21% (23)

Age: ranged from 31 to 73 years with the majority aged 40 to 70. One might question why people in their 60s and 70s are being rehabilitated. Longevity is increasing, and many elderly patients are very active. Some of the 70-year-old people are much more active physically with regard to dancing, golfing, and various daily living activities, than are the younger patients.

Medical: 53 myocardial infarction and stable angina

Surgical: 60 coronary artery bypass surgery and heart valve replacements

No major complications have occurred during the exercise sessions. Of the 113, 6 patients have died; 2 deaths were coronary related:

2 from preexisting carcinoma

1 from cerebral bleeding after a stroke

1 from pulmonary edema

1 suddenly at home during sleep

1 arrested at home

Description of Program

First, there is a two day functional evaluation which includes the following:

Blood work

Chest x-ray

Pulmonary function test

Echocardiogram

24-hour holter monitor

Minnesota multiphasic personality test (psychological test)

Graded exercise tolerance test

Cardiac exam

Assessment interviews are conducted by team members, including a dietitian, exercise physiologist, and cardiac nurse. The interviews are designed to determine the patient's level of knowledge, concerns, needs, and goals.

The three-month program consists of one hour of exercise on telemetry and one hour of group discussion three times per week for two months. During the last month, the patients come once a week. The patients are reevaluated at the end of three months. All tests are repeated, and the patients discuss their situations individually with the physician and in a group meeting with the nurse, exercise physiologist, and dietitian. Patients may voluntarily return once a week to exercise. The voluntary exercise compliance allows for continuing assessment of the patients' ongoing health status.

Components of the Program

The philosophy of the program is that a multidisciplinary approach best meets the patients' needs. There are frequent meetings to discuss the patients and program strategies, which are individually developed to best help them meet their specific goals. Once a week, all of the cardiologists meet with the team to discuss the patients' progress. Team members attend all of the group discussions which focus on the patient's status.

The program consists of first, an exercise program; second, an educational component in which there are group meetings and one-to-one counseling with a nurse, exercise physiologist, or dietitian whenever needed; and, third, a medical component, which means that a patient is seen by a physician should any problems arise.

The Exercise Component

The exercise component of the rehabilitation program is founded on specific information pertinent to the development and implementation of a highly personalized exercise prescription. Prior to meeting with the program participant, and, hopefully, the spouse or significant other, all of the patient's available medical records are scrutinized along with the program's battery of physiologic evaluations. Historically, the focus is on the patient's age, education, occupation, previous medical history, and cardiac risk factors. Somatically, particular attention is paid to the participant's graded exercise evaluation, echocardiogram, catheterization report, operative and postoperative course, and pulmonary function results.

After digesting all of the above material, team members discuss with the patient and spouse their previous and current life styles, their existing concerns and future aspirations, their preventive health-care concepts, as well as any questions they may have regarding the rehabilitation program, particularly the exercise aspect. Personally, the team stresses above all else that the patients are thought of as human beings rather than as neutered medical entities. The program is one of mutual trust and friendship, and team members emphatically feel that these attributes are essential to any successful rehabilitation endeavor.

Clinically, a multistation interval-training approach is utilized. The multistation application is purposely designed to improve the functional capacity of the patients' arms and legs. The patient's upper torso is exercised since consistently most patients complain of markedly diminished upper-body strength. This lack of strength translates into a negative psychologic outlook which tends to limit the patients' performance of various daily living and recreational activities.

The interval-training format allows a significant proportion of the patient population to initially perform more exercise, to improve their cardiovascular fitness in a gradual yet progressive manner, and to minimize muscle soreness. This format also places all of the exercise equipment at the patient's disposal. Psychologically, the interval-training format fosters greater patient-to-patient communication and patient-to-staff interaction, and it helps to lessen the patient's subjective level of perceived exertion, thereby placing the exercise in a more enjoyable light. All of these positive variables play a major role in enhancing patient camaraderie and program compliance.

The exercise program consists of three distinct periods: the warm-up, training, and cool-down periods. For example, during the warm-up period, patients cycle for four minutes, take their own pulse, then dismount and walk at a normal pace for two minutes. The same format is followed when the patients cool down. The training period consists of the patients varying their exercise (arm-leg) again for four minutes before taking their pulse and walking for two minutes for six repetitions. Blood pressures are taken before, during, and after exercise. The patients use all of the equipment and a large percentage of their total muscle mass.

One cardinal rule that is followed without exemption is that of not allowing the patients to perform back-to-back upper-body exercises. The team wants to negate the possibility of a rapid, sustained, overtly high systolic blood pressure response while minimizing the patients' subjective feelings of fatigue and discomfort via increasing lactate levels.

The initial length of the patient's program is based on recent convalescence, complicated or noncomplicated, phase one and home exercise activities, graded exercise evaluations, and the team's subjective perception of presenting physiognomy. Ideally, the end point of a patient's program, excluding the five-minute warm-up and cool-down periods, is thirty minutes at hemodynamicaly appropriate intensity. The thirty minutes are usually subdivided into 6 five-minute intervals of varied arm and leg movements interspersed with 2-minute walk segments. Most of the patients are gradually able to reach the ideal maximal exercise duration.

Generally, the patients' exercise intensities are predicted on their preprogram graded exercise-tolerance heart rate and blood pressure response. The younger, uncomplicated, recently active, postaortocoronary bypass patients are usually exercised at a higher initial intensity, that is, 80% to 85% of peak graded exercise test double product. Conversely, the older, more complicated, less active, myocardial infarct-bypass patients are begun at a lower intensity; that is, 65% to 75% of peak graded exercise test double product. The double product of the latter group is usually elevated over a three- to five-week period. In a few cases, the team continues to exercise patients at the lower intensity throughout the program.

On the extreme ends are two nonconformist exercise responders. First is the subgroup of those who are unable to elevate their exercise double products to the level of their preprogram graded exercise test figures. Leg fatigue, respiratory distress, and increased dosages of beta-blocking agents are usually the prime predisposing factors associated with the seemingly incongruent chronotropic-blood pressure response. The second subgroup are those patients who show little difference between the resting and peak exercise double products. These patients are usually older, more functionally infirm, and highly medicated, or they are younger patients who have a low pain threshold, are poorly motivated, and have significant muscle weakness. Whichever the case, the strategy was amended by placing a greater emphasis on patient observation and perceived exertion when developing the exercise prescription. In summary, the phase 2 exercise program is a multistationed, interval-training approach that is individualized, flexible, beneficial, and safe. The statistical results have been gratifying, while the humanistic interaction has been spiritually uplifting.

Bibliography

American Heart Association. *Cardiac Rehabilitation Unit Program Guide,* American Heart Association, October 1977.
———*Coronary Care: Rehabilitation after Myocardial Infarction.* Dallas: American Heart Association, 1973.
———*Directory of Cardiac Rehabilitation Units 1975–1976.* American Heart Association.
———*Exercise Standards Book.* Dallas: American Heart Association, 1979.
Clausen, T.P. Circulatory adjustments to dynamic exercise and effect of physical training in normal subjects and in patients with coronary artery disease. *Prog. Cardiovas. Dis.* 18:459–495, 1976.
Clausen, T.P., Klausen, K., Rasmussen, B., and Trap-Jensen, T. Central and peripheral circulatory changes after training of the arms or legs. *Am. J. Physiol.* 225:675–682, 1973.
Kavanagh, T. *Heart Attack?—Counter Attack.* Toronto: Van Nostrand Reinhold Ltd., 1976.
Leon, A.S., and Blackburn, H. Exercise rehabilitation of the coronary heart disease patient. *Geriatrics* 32:66–76, 1977.
Pollock, M.L. The quantification of endurance training program. In J. Wilmore (Ed.), *Exercise and Sports Sciences Reviews,* Vol. One, New York: Academic Press, 1973.
Rowell, L. Human cardiovascular adjustments to exercise and thermal stress. *Physiol. Rev.* 54:75–159, 1974.
Sanne, H. Exercise tolerance and physical training of non-selected patients after myocardial infarction. *Acta. Scand. Med.* (suppl. 5511):1–124, 1973.
Schuer, J., and Tipton, C.M. Cardiovascular adaptations to physical training. *Annu. Rev. Physiol.* 39:221–251, 1977.
Wenger, N.K., and Hellerstein, H.K. *Rehabilitation of the Coronary Patient.* New York: Wiley Medical Publication, 1978.

11 Community-Based Cardiac Rehabilitation

Catherine Certo, R.P.T., M.S.

In the late 1960s Herman Hellerstein, a cardiologist, designed an exercise program for his patients in a local community center. The original objective of his program was to determine whether a physical conditioning program, located outside of the usual medical model, could provide the basic physiologic, psychologic, vocational, and personal aspects seen in most inpatient programs. This program was an outstanding success. Later it was moved to the local YMCA. In each case, supervision of the program was the dual responsibility of the physician and well-informed physical health educators working in collaboration.

In the case of Dr. Hellerstein, the outpatient community-based programs were an outgrowth of the already successful inpatient cardiac rehabilitation programs provided by cardiologists such as Dr. Lenore Zohman and Dr. Nanette Wenger. However, in the Boston area in the late 1960s and early 1970s, inpatient cardiac rehabilitation was not very successful. Most hospitals were conservative in their approach to cardiac patients even though there was a growing consensus that physical inactivity was detrimental for coronary patients. Upon discharge, patients were given the suggestion that they might go to the local YMCA and become involved in a program of walking and moderate calisthenics. Driven by fear and the desire to beat the odds, many of these coronary patients in the Boston area began to join local YMCAs. The YMCAs provided exercise leaders and a modest range of calisthenics. In an effort to provide these patients with a program that was safe and effective, the Cambridge YMCA in 1971 began an outpatient cardiac rehabilitation program under the medical supervision of L. Howard Hartley, M.D. This was Boston's first cardiac rehabilitation program. Many inpatient programs and outpatient hospital-based programs followed this trend in the next several years. By the end of 1977, there was such a demand for outpatient programs that the Brockton YMCA began a cardiac rehabilitation program followed shortly thereafter by the Boston YMCA.

Since it started nearly a decade ago, it is clear that the community-based program is not new to the Boston area. What is new is the community-based program located at Northeastern University. This program is a year and a half old, and it is the first university-based program in the Boston area. This program is similar to those located at the University of Wisconsin at

LaCrosse and at Wake Forest. The program is designed to serve the greater Boston business and medical communities as well as to provide an educational experience for health and exercise professionals. Undergraduates as well as graduate students can gain firsthand experience as exercise technologists, exercise leaders, health counselors, physical therapists, and researchers.

The purpose of the cardiac rehabilitation program is to provide a comprehensive medical and therapeutic program for those individuals with coronary heart disease or those who are at high risk of developing this disease. The goal of the program is to help these patients reestablish themselves physiologically, emotionally, and socially after discharge from a hospital or an outpatient rehabilitation program.

The staff includes a cardiologist, a physical therapist, a cardiac nurse, and certified exercise leaders. Their primary objective is to assist the patients during their period of adjustment and rehabilitation. In this program, the physical therapist is responsible for executing the patient's prescribed patient education and emergency care.

The medical evaluation includes a cardiopulmonary examination including a detailed medical history review, a graded treadmill test using the Balke protocol, blood pressure evaluation, blood lipid profile, pulmonary function tests, personality and stress-related behavioral inventories, medication profile, coronary risk factor profile, and an exercise prescription.

The population includes post-myocardial infarction patients, post-coronary bypass or valvular surgery patients at approximately eight to ten weeks following hospitalization, and individuals with documented coronary artery disease or with high risk of coronary artery disease.

At this time, the program is not receiving reimbursement from third-party insurance carriers. While there have been negotiations with Blue Cross-Blue Shield, to date they are not covering the program's services. However, some of the patients individually have received reimbursement up to 80%. This, of course, depends on the type of policy one is carrying. The program provides an itemized bill for the exercise stress test as well as each of the exercise sessions. This in turn can be used by the subscribers as a bill to submit to their insurance companies.

Each one-hour exercise class includes a fifteen-minute warm-up exercise period. This is especially helpful to those patients who have not exercised for a long period of time. It also serves to alleviate low back strain, as specific exercises are included to increase abdominal strength and hamstring flexibility. This is followed by twenty to thirty minutes of walking, jogging, or bicycle activity, followed by ten minutes of warm-down and relaxation exercises. Each participant's exercise program is individually prescribed, based on the results of the initial evaluation and exercise-perceived exertion tests conducted in the gymnasium with ECG monitoring. Following an orientation period with continuous monitoring, each participant is monitored once a week or more frequently if warranted. The objective is the gradual withdrawal from the dependence on monitoring for most patients, while maintaining a safe exercise commitment.

Most patients prefer group programs where physical activity is varied. Patients either learn or relearn to perform a regimen of calisthenics or intermittent walk/jog sequence or to play games. For the patients, the program has instituted either basketball or volleyball once a week.

These activities provide the stimulus for participation because they are not physically exhausting, give patients the opportunity to play at their own levels of capability, and at the same time provide a healthy competitive spirit which promotes individual and group interaction.

Weekly health education seminars offer assistance to individuals who embark upon personal commitment to lifelong exercise and improved health habits. The faculty conduct discussions on topics such as:

Coronary artery disease and its risk

Role of exercise in cardiovascular health and disease

Nutrition and cardiovascular health

Diet and weight reduction

Stress, personality type, and cardiovascular health

Stress management

Smoking cessation

Sexuality and the cardiac patient

Cardiopulmonary resuscitation

After each exercise session, a specific topic of interest is discussed. The weekly health seminars often serve as a catalyst for small group discussion. During this time, the cardiac-care nurse personally offers assistance to individuals who feel they may need additional assistance. Clinical observations have long recognized that the psychologic problems which face the cardiac patient can be overwhelming. These include anxiety, fear of sudden death, the lack of self-confidence. The program has seen tremendous psychologic gains in cardiac patients involved in exercise programs. This profit can be interpreted as an increase in emotional stability as participants see an improvement in their physical capabilities. Participants can and should be encouraged to include spouses, family members, and significant others in many program activities.

The success of long-term exercise programs for cardiac patients is measured by adherence and the improvement of the patient. Consequently, participants need to be assessed regularly, and such improvement needs to be shared with the patients and their physicians. For most of the patients, this is done once a month using telemetry. The results are discussed with the patient, and the ECG strips along with the new exercise prescription are forwarded to the personal physician.

Most of the patients stay six months in the program. Then they are retested and given an exercise prescription. At this point, several options are offered to the patient. With the approval of the cardiologist, some patients may be admitted to the regular Adult Fitness Program and eventually may join the Jogging Club. Those who need more supervision but are unable to come in on a regular basis are given a home program and return once a month for reevaluation of the prescription.

As Dr. Michael Sach pointed out in chapter 3, "Three major components are needed for successful programs, the group setting, the convenience of the program, and the support." The community-based program at Northeastern sincerely attempts to provide these three basic components for its participants and it strongly seeks the support of physicians and surgeons.

V   Sports Injuries

12 Upper-Extremity Injuries: Overuse Syndromes of the Shoulder

Arthur L. Boland, M.D.

Although traumatic upper-extremity injuries remain very significant problems for athletes, there has been a recent increase in the troublesome overuse syndromes involving the shoulder region. The painful pitcher's shoulder has plagued participants, trainers, and team physicians for years, and now similar chronic injuries are frequently seen among recreational as well as competitive swimmers and tennis enthusiasts. Insidious in onset and only annoying in the initial stages, these injuries may relentlessly increase in intensity and severity and may eventually totally disable the athlete. This chapter will discuss some of the anatomical factors peculiar to this region to review diagnostic and therapeutic steps needed for their management and prevention.

Anatomy

The shoulder is a complex region consisting of the glenohumeral joint, its static capsular support, and the dynamic muscle groups which control the motion of the shoulder girdle. The shoulder has the widest range of motion of any joint in the body. Normal function at the sternoclavicular joint, the acromioclavicular joint, and along the scapular thoracic plane are essential for full activity of the upper extremity.

The humeral head articulates with a relatively small biconcave glenoid fossa. The humeral head faces medially, superiorly, and approximately 30 degrees posteriorly. The glenoid which has a surface area only approximately one-third that of the humeral head is directed anteriorly, laterally, and slightly superiorly. The cartilaginous glenoid labrum adds additional support to the joint. The angulation of the glenohumeral joint, therefore, makes the humeral head more unstable anteriorly, The acromion and the coracoacromial ligament protects the joint superiorly. Shoulder abduction and elevation depend upon motion through the sternoclavicular and acromioclavicular joints. The acromioclavicular joint moves in vertical, frontal and horizontal axes while the scapula rotates and elevates along the thoracic wall. The coracoclavicular ligaments (conoid and trapezoid ligaments) limit the amount of motion through the acromioclavicular joint.

The capsule of the shoulder joint lends static support to the glenohumeral joint. The coracohumeral ligament extends across the superior aspect of the capsule, and thickened areas within the capsule anteriorly are referred to as the glenohumeral ligaments. The inferior and middle portions of the glenohumeral capsule are particularly important in restraining the humeral head during abduction and external rotation. The muscle groups around the shoulder girdle are very complex and must work in a coordinated fashion to produce smooth motion of the joint. The rotator cuff muscles, the subscapularis anteriorly, the supraspinatous superiorly, and the infraspinatous and teres minor posteriorly blend with the capsule and attach into the proximal humerus. The biceps tendon extends from the glenoid through the joint superiorly and into the bicipital groove between the greater and lesser tuberosities of the humerus. Scapular elevation and adduction are controlled by the trapezius, levator scapulae, and rhomboid muscle groups. The serratus anterior, which attaches to the inferior pole of the scapula, assists in scapular rotation. The triceps and coracobrachialis muscles, as well as the biceps, traverse the shoulder joint area and extend down the upper arm. The pectoral muscles and latissimus dorsi muscle, originating from the rib cage anteriorly and posteriorly respectively, attach into the proximal humerus and help control forward flexion and extension. The contributions these different muscles make about the shoulder vary depending on the position of the arm at any one time. A complete understanding of the functional anatomy of the shoulder is essential in diagnosing the painful shoulder.

An overuse syndrome is defined as a chronic inflammatory condition caused by repeated microtrauma from a repetitious activity. Blazina originally classified these injuries into first degree or those causing pain only after activity; second degree, those producing pain during participation and after but not sufficient to interfere with performance; and third degree injuries which resulted in disabling pain both during and after participation [4].

Overuse syndromes around the shoulder are particularly common in throwing sports, swimming, and in tennis. In order to appreciate the spectrum of injuries which may occur in throwing, one must comprehend the mechanism of this strenuous activity. King and colleagues have classified the phases of throwing and pointed out those structures which participate in each step [9]. During the initial cocking motion, the arm is brought back into abduction, extension, and external rotation. Consequently, the middle and posterior aspects of the deltoid are functioning as well as the infraspinatous and teres minor to produce rotation. The trapezius and rhomboids contribute to scapular elevation and adduction. During the cocking stage, the posterior capsule is relaxed, whereas the anterior capsule, subscapularis, and pectoral muscles are passively elongating. The next stage of throwing consists of the acceleration phase in which the arm begins to move forward again, often preceded by a forward rotation of the trunk. During this activity, the anterior muscle groups, particularly the subscapularis, pectorals, and anterior deltoid, are contracting while still lengthening (eccentrically). The biceps muscle also may contract increasing tension on the tendon within the bicipital groove which is externally rotated. It is during this early part of the accleration phase that the anterior capsule is particularly stretched. As the arm comes forward into the final follow-through position, the posterior capsule and external rotators are relaxed and passively stretched. Other authors have enumerated the various shoulder lesions which can occur during throwing [10–13]. Anteriorly the capsular ligaments can become attenuated and allow the humeral head to sublux and even dislocate. Sudden contractures of the subscapularis and pectoral muscles can produce tearing and rupture of these muscular tendinous units. Impingement can occur anteriorly around the coracoid and also posteriorly as the humeral head abuts on the glenoid. The bicipital tendon and supraspinatous tendon can abut on the acromion and coracoacromial ligament producing impingement syndromes. Small tears in the rotator cuff muscles as well as chronic subdeltoid bursitis frequently follow as a result of these repeated impingements. Bennett has described hypertrophic bony changes along the inferior aspect of the glenoid [2], and King et al. have reported chronic subluxation of the biceps tendon from its groove [9]. Since the acromioclavicular joint contributes to abduction and rotation, chronic degenerative changes at that site may produce pain felt over the top of the shoulder and radiating both anteriorly and posteriorly. It is obvious that the throwing mechanism is very complex and can cause symptoms in numerous areas. A great deal of diligence is required in questioning and examining these patients in order to determine the site of the pathology.

Priest and Nagel have recently reviewed shoulder injuries in tennis players [14]. It has been pointed out that the overhead serve is quite similar to a throwing motion and produces many of the same injuries that we see in pitchers.

Kennedy and Hawkins have defined a condition referred to as swimmer's shoulder [6]. Both the freestyle and butterfly strokes produce repeated impingement of the greater tuberosity under the coracoacromial arch. As the arm is brought forward into abduction, forward flexion, and internal rotation, the region of the supraspinatous tendon and biceps tendon in its groove sustain repeated trauma under the acromion and coracoacromial ligament. As the arm is then pulled down into an abducted position in the follow-through motion, the blood flow into the distal portion of the rotator cuff and biceps tendon is impeded by the pressure of the humeral head from below. MacNab and Rathburn demonstrated these areas of avascularity in their microvascular studies of the rotator cuff [11].

Diagnosis

A careful history is perhaps the most important step in making the diagnosis of overuse syndromes. A previous history of shoulder subluxation or an acromioclavicular joint separation should be pursued. One must be familiar with the patient's previous training program. These injuries are frequently seen early in the season and often during periods of double-session workouts. Repeated examinations are often necessary to localize the site of the tenderness and particularly to detect relative weaknesses in the rotator muscle groups. A complete neurological examination is needed to rule out cervical radiculitis, entrapment of the suprascapular or axillary nerves, as well as thoracic outlet syndromes. Vascular problems in the subclavium and brachial systems must also be considered.

Routine x-rays, including the Westpoint view to demonstrate the glenoid, should be obtained. Exostoses along the anterior and inferior aspects of the glenoid may require special views. Degenerative changes at the acromioclavicular joint must also be ruled out. Shoulder arthrograms may be indicated when a rotator cuff tear is suspected. An enlarged capsule may also be noted on arthrography in a chronic subluxing shoulder. Jackson has pointed out that chronic impingement syndromes produce thickening and contraction of the subdeltoid bursa [5]. He has performed bursagrams which nicely illustrate this problem. These additional x-ray studies should be done only after a careful examination has been performed to determine the exact site of tenderness, the arc of motion which produces pain, and the presence of any specific weakness.

Treatment

Treatment of these overuse syndromes is directed at reducing inflammation and also altering training and performance techniques to prevent recurrence. The type 1 and type 2 injuries, which produce pain primarily after participation and are not disabling, should be treated promptly to prevent their progression. Proper warm-up prior to participation and then ice following competition may help to relieve the inflammatory changes. Oral anti-inflammatory agents such as aspirin or one of the other nonsteroidal medications are often helpful. Reducing the amount of time throwing, swimming, or serving may help to control the pain. It is essential to review the problem with the coach since minor changes in technique such as the amount of elevation in the arm in throwing or swimming may be necessary. Since these injuries frequently lead to contracture and muscle weakness, it is essential to seek these problems out and correct them with flexibility exercises and specific strengthening programs. The isokinetic machines are very helpful in detecting relative weaknesses about the shoulder.

The third degree injuries usually require a period of rest. During this time conditioning programs for the other areas of the body may be continued. Local injections of steroids into the involved areas have been helpful in some cases. However, it must be remembered that these injections produce local tissue necrosis and weaken the structures for at least two weeks. During that time no vigorous participation should be undertaken. Other modalities can be used to reduce inflammation, especially ultrasound and diathermy. Since recurrence of these injuries is very common, the participant must have full range of motion, equal strength, and be pain free before returning to competition. Since both coordination and endurance are essential in these sports, it is important to progress the rehabilitation program slowly to avoid future difficulties.

References

1. Barnes, D.A., and Tullos, H.S. An analysis of 100 symptomatic baseball players. *AJSM* 6, no. 2:62–69, 1978.

2. Bennett, G.E. Shoulder and elbow lesions of the professional baseball pitcher. *JAMA* 117:510–514, 1941.

3. Bennett, G.E. Shoulder and elbow lesions distinctive of baseball players. *Am. Surg.* 126:107, 1947.

4. Blazina, M.E., Jumper's knee. *Orthop. Clin. North Am.* 4:665–678, 1973.

5. Jackson, D.W. Chronic rotator cuff impingement in the throwing athlete. *AJSM* 4, no. 6:231, 1976.

6. Kennedy, J.C., and Hawkins, P.T. Swimmer's shoulder. *Phys. Sports Med.* 2:35–38, 1974.

7. Kennedy, J.C., Hawkins, R., and Kressoff, W.B. Orthopedic manifestations of swimming. *AJSM* 6, no. 6:309–322, 1978.

8. Kennedy, J.C., and Willis, R.B. The effects of local steroid injections on tendons: A biomechanical and microscopic correlative study. *Am. J. Sports Med.* 4:11–21, 1976.

9. King, J.W., Brelsford, H.J., and Tullos, H.S. Analysis of the pitching arm of the professional baseball pitcher. *Clin. Ortho.* 67:116, 1969.

10. Lombardo, S.J., Jobe, F.W., Kerlan, R., et al. Posterior shoulder lesions in throwing athletes. *AJSM* 5, no. 3:106–110, 1977.

11. MacNab, I., and Rathburn, J.B. The microvascular pattern of the rotator cuff. *JBJS* 52B:524–527, 1970.

12. Neer, C.S. Anterior acromioplasty for chronic impingement syndrome in the shoulder. *JBJS* 54A:41–50, 1972.

13. Norwood, L.A., Del Pizzo, W., Jobe, F.W., and Kerlan, R.K. Anterior shoulder pain in baseball pitchers. *AJSM* 6, no. 3:103–105, 1978.

14. Priest, J.D., and Nagel, D.A. Tennis shoulder. *AJSM* 4 (1):28–42, 1976.

15. Richardson, A.B., Jobe, F.W., and Collins, R.H. The shoulder in competitive swimming. *AJSM* 8, no. 3:159, 1980.

13 Lower-Extremity Injuries: Overuse Injuries in the Recreational Adult

Lyle J. Micheli, M.D.

It is evident to even the most casual observer that this country is in the midst of a fitness explosion. American men, women, and children of all ages, sizes, and shapes are turning to activities as diverse as jogging, racquetball, and roller skating for exercise and recreation. Increased leisure time and changed attitudes toward youth, aging, and the social roles of men and women have provided the foundations for this movement. Increased emphasis on exercise in weight loss programs, suggested relationships between regular exercise and longevity or even productivity, and improved psychic states have provided further stimulus to many a new jogger or athlete [2].

Whatever the motivation, these new or renewed athletes and fitness enthusiasts are presenting physicians with a new set of problems and questions. In the more traditional sports medicine setting, the injured athlete presented himself to the team doctor, often at the direction of, or at least with the approval of, the coach. If the team was fortunate enough to have an athletic trainer, the athlete may have had an initial assessment by the trainer before seeing the doctor. The team doctor's primary role was to confirm the diagnosis, estimate the severity of the injury, and, most importantly, prognosticate return to action in conjunction with an appropriate treatment and rehabilitation program. In the design of a particular rehabilitation program for an athlete in a particular sport, the team doctor could usually count heavily on the resources of coach and trainer for supervision and progression.

Recreational Sports Medicine

Lacking coach, trainer, and often knowledge of either fundamentals of fitness training or even playing skills in the new sport, the recreational athlete's most accessible resource is often the physician dealing with the sports injury. While at first exposure, questions about running shoes, running surface, type of tennis racquet or ski binding, or even recommended types of hockey helmets or face masks may be both baffling and apparently inappropriate questions for a doctor, studies of a number of sports and their injuries confirm the importance of such factors in the occurrence and severity of sports injuries [11].

121

It is this aspect of sports-related injuries—the potential for decreasing the incidence or severity of injury by appropriate prevention and careful rehabilitation—that makes sports medicine a separate discipline. Much of the controversy and confusion about this field appears unwarranted and unnecessary if sports medicine is seen primarily as a field of preventive medicine, analogous to industrial or environmental medicine, where every effort is made to determine the host and environmental risk factors in each sport or recreational activity and then to institute changes which will decrease the occurrence or severity of injury [3]. While the therapeutics of sports injuries are important, they remain secondary to determining the risk and decreasing the incidence or severity of injuries in sports.

Sports and recreational activities are particularly amenable to this approach. The rules, duration of exposure, equipment, and participant selection in sports are, of their very nature, arbitrary and changeable. While certain conditions in the factory, marketplace, or environment may be changed only with great difficulty, one can more easily require protective helmets for hockey or horseback riding, disallow cross-body blocking in children's football, or curve-ball throwing in children's baseball [6].

One might agree with the critics who indignantly claim that the treatment of a fractured wrist in a football player or an Achilles tendinitis in a runner differs little from those occurring in nonathletes and should not be defined as the special prerogative of a sports doctor. However, any physician who deals with athletes and their injuries should have a particular interest in assessing the environment in which they occur and determining means of prevention as well as taking steps to prevent reinjury.

It would appear that the primary justification for this discipline rests on its potential for the use of epidemiologic methods in order to decrease the incidence in sports and recreation. Providing special treatment for professional or Olympic athletes, while perhaps of importance economically or politically, would appear a rather weak justification for the development of a separate medical care system. Determining the risks and benefits of sports activities in order to prevent sports injuries and to use sports to improve health would appear a much sounder justification.

Overuse Injuries

The growth in numbers of recreational athletes has been paralleled by a growing awareness by physicians of a heterogenous collection of injuries which have begun to be grouped together because they share a common mechanism of injury: repetitive microtrauma. Repetitive microtrauma, as in striking the foot against the ground in running, is usually superimposed upon a combination of other factors, such as anatomic malalignment or training errors, and results in tissue injury [1].

The more traditional mechanism of injury, a single episode of macro-trauma, such as a cross-body block in football or a twisting fall in skiing, has resulted in the more traditional sports injuries: sprains of ligaments, contusions or bruises of muscle, and fractures of bones—the impact injuries. It has been less usual to consider the impact of the foot against the ground in running or striking a ball with a tennis racquet as trauma, yet these innocuous impacts, particularly if done too frequently over too short a period of time, can tear muscles and tendons, destroy articular cartilage, and fracture bones.

Types of Injuries

Every major tissue of the musculo-skeletal system is subject to overuse injuries. In the muscle-tendon units, the major overuse injury is tendinitis; through muscle strains the results of microtrauma of muscle tissue or supporting tissue can be seen. It is important to remember that the inflammatory phase of tendinitis with heat, swelling, pain, and erythema is really the body's normal initial healing response to injured tissue, and this response must be respected, or one will suffer the consequences. While it is rarely necessary to totally discontinue the use of an injured extremity, and complete rest may actually delay the healing, a period of relative rest during which the extremity is used, but with a different stress pattern, may be required. A runner with an acute Achilles tendinitis who is swimming five miles a day may not be running, but he or she is certainly not resting.

It is important to maintain the strength and flexibility of a muscle-tendon unit while one is recovering from an acute tendinitis. Pain and swelling are good guides to the limits of training; icing and gentle compression are often invaluable aids in maintaining conditioning during the recovery phase. Some recent work from Dalhousie University in Halifax, Nova Scotia suggests that dynamic eccentric work can safely be done with a muscle-tendon unit tendinitis and may actually speed up healing [10]. In ligamentous tissue, bursitis is the major overuse injury. A bursa is actually only a potential space in which adjunct tissues, such as ligaments and tendons, sustain irritation and injury.

The overuse injury of bone is, of course, stress fracture or fatigue fracture. Although most often seen in the long bones of the lower leg, tibia, and fibula, it is the great masquerader. In any persistent, activity-related extremity pain, whether of foot, hip, knee, or ankle, stress fracture must be suspected. During a seven-month period in the sports medicine clinic of Children's Hospital, a total of 53 stress fractures of the lower extremity were diagnosed, including five hip fractures [8]. Again, in ballet dancers persistent foot pain, often initially diagnosed as tendinitis or metatarsalgia, will often be finally determined to be a stress fracture. This diagnosis can be very difficult to make by physical examination or even x-ray, and Te^{99} bone scan may be necessary for final confirmation.

In articular cartilage, repetitive microtrauma appears to result in a pattern of injury starting with softening, and it can progress to shredding and thinning of the articular surface down to the underlying bone. The characteristic history of activity-related aching type pain in the front of the knee, increased by climbing stairs and, ironically, by prolonged sitting with the knees bent (called the movie sign), is usually helpful in making the diagnosis.

Associated Risk Factors

Most of the information and impressions concerning additional factors which may predispose to injury come from the assessments of athletes who have sustained overuse injuries. From this review has come a checklist of risk factors for overuse injury which has been found useful when evaluating an athlete for steps to be taken in preventing the occurrence or reoccurrence of injury.

1. Training errors including abrupt changes in intensity, duration, or frequency of training
2. Musculotendinous imbalance of strength, flexibility, or bulk
3. Anatomical malalignment of the lower extremities, including differences in leg lengths, abnormalities of rotation of the hips, position of the kneecap, and bow legs, knock knees, or flat feet
4. Footwear: improper fit, inadequate impact-absorbing material, excessive stiffness of the sole, and/or insufficient support of hindfoot
5. Running surface: concrete pavement versus asphalt, versus running track, versus dirt or grass
6. Associated disease state of the lower extremity, including arthritis, poor circulation, old fracture or other injury

This checklist has proven useful in approaching overuse injuries in a variety of activities including running, dance, gymnastics, and even diving. For dance, technique must be added as an additional risk factor.

It is noteworthy that sex of participant is not on the list. While it appears at present that the new female runner may be sustaining a higher incidence of overuse injuries than similar groups of males by age, this truly appears to be a cultural phenomenon, the result of significantly less running as teen-agers by girls, and can really be classed as a training error. This was especially true for a group of culturally deconditioned women begun on running programs designed for men, as seen early on in female military academy entrants [7].

While increases in cardiovascular fitness can safely be attained in a matter of months, the time course of musculo-skeletal conditioning and strengthening, particularly of the bones, may be much slower. These tissues may take much longer to remodel and strengthen themselves for increased physical demands, particularly if underutilized for a number of years.

Experience with sports injuries in the female suggests that, although the rate of injury in certain female sports, such as running, may be higher than in similar male programs at their initiation, this rate progressively decreases as time goes on. An example comes to mind. Four years ago, when women first began to play rugby football in the Boston area, the rate of overuse injuries from running training alone in these new ruggers was surprisingly high and was actually greater than the impact injuries sustained in this vigorous contact sport. This year overuse injuries in these athletes are at a minimum, reflecting progressive improvement in the fitness level of these players as well as a more appropriate matching of training rate and intensity.

It is important to remember that certain sports, if done exclusively, may actually contribute to muscle-tendon imbalances. Running, if done exclusively, tends to tighten and strengthen low back muscles and fascia as well as the quadriceps muscles and calf muscles and results in a relative imbalance with their opposing muscles. If supplemental flexibility exercises are not also done, this muscle-tendon imbalance can predispose one to back, hip, knee, and lower-leg injuries.

Anatomic malalignment can be the risk factor for which it is most difficult to compensate. If a dancer begins to suffer knee pain and injuries because the hips lack sufficient turnout or external rotation for a technically satisfactory plie, little can be done. Similarly, runners lacking rotation about the hips, particularly internal rotation, may never be able to run without a repetitive pattern of injuries and might be counseled to consider biking or swimming.

On the other hand, some rather dynamic malalignments about the knee, lower leg, or foot may be completely compatible with injury-free participation. Some of the most effective runners have dramatic lower-leg bowing and run without problems. Similarly, flat or pronated feet are often indicated as a major factor in the occurrence of lower-extremity overuse injury, and yet a number of world class runners and premier dancers have severely pronated feet and function without problem. In other athletes, however, compensation for these alignments can sometimes be done with orthotic inserts in the shoes. The use of these devices in the management of knee and lower-leg problems in some athletes has been especially successful [4].

Thus, it must be evident that it is truly a combination of factors that results in a given overuse injury in a given athlete. In the study of stress fractures noted previously, training error was the most prevalent risk factor associated with the occurrence of injury, followed closely by muscle-tendon imbalance and anatomic malalignment.

It is important to recognize that overuse injury is not seen only in the recreational or less skilled athlete. A nationally ranked runner who had been training at more than ninety miles a week dropped below seventy miles during a three-week examination period and then immediately resumed his ninety mile pace. A stress fracture of the tibia resulted, somewhat to his embarrassment. Additional risk factors appeared to be the use of a worn pair of racing flats from the previous season and tight calf muscles.

Sites of Injury

With this preview of the types of injury and associated risk factors, it should still be useful to review the anatomic sites of injury and discuss the injuries most frequently seen at each site. Low back pain can be a distressing overuse injury, particularly in the runner. As noted previously, running tends to tighten the posterior low back muscles and fascia. The resulting tendency to low back sway or lordosis increases the risk for a number of low back conditions, including ruptured disc, facet syndrome, and spondylolysis. Supplemental low back and hamstring stretching and abdominal stengthening are the first step in injury prevention [5].

Overuse injuries about the hip include trochanteric bursitis, ileopsoas tendinitis, and, although frequently unsuspected, stress fractures. In trochanteric bursitis, tight fascia lata and hamstrings as well as minor leg length discrepancies (the bursitis usually occurs in the longer leg) are frequently associated risk factors.

The most frequent overuse injury about the knee, as already noted is chondromalacia or patello-femoral stress syndrome. In addition, lateral knee pain can frequently be encountered in runners. This may be unilateral or bilateral and has a high association with the anatomic malalignment of genu valgum and tibia vara. Again, long leg syndrome also can be seen with unilateral lateral knee pain. A number of anatomic structures and conditions have been indicated as the cause of this pain, including popliteal tendinitis, impingement of the fascia lata on the lateral femoral condyle, and chondromalacia of the patella. This lateral knee pain appears to be one of the conditions which can be helped by orthotics in the shoes. Again, relative training error is often seen as an associated risk factor in overuse knee pain. Tight hamstrings should also be watched for in these syndromes.

A program of static straight-leg-raising exercises done with progressive resistance and combined with lower-extremity flexibility exercise, has helped to solve this problem. A recent survey of young patients with patello-femoral stress syndrome showed than more than 90% of them were cleared of pain and resumed function with this program. It is interesting to observe that the ability to lift 12 pounds ten times with straight leg appears to be a threshold. Patients who reach this will almost always have a satisfactory result with an overall program of six months of exercise. The goal for lifting is generally between 18 and 25 pounds, done with three sets of 10 on each leg.

In the lower leg, various tendinitides are seen with great frequency as overuse injuries. Once again, an index of suspicion must be maintained for stress fracture. Recently, Puddu and others have called attention to tendinosis or aseptic necrosis of tendon tissue as an additional cause of dysfunction and pain in major tendons, including the Achilles tendon [9]. These sites undergo ischemic death, much as can occur in bone, and are not successfully healed and revascularized by the body. Continued pain, and in some cases, complete tendon rupture may result if significant mechanical compromise has occurred.

The important risk factors in these cases appear to be inflexibility of musculo-tendon units and, often, training error, repetitive in nature. Perhaps the single most important preventive step is daily slow stretching, particularly of the Achilles, and maintenance of the dorsiflexor strength by heel walking or resistive exercises.

One of the most difficult overuse injuries of all occurs in the foot, plantar facsitis. The plantar fascia is a heavy layer of tissue running from the front of the heel bone, or os calcis, to the base of the metacarpo-phalangeal joints along the arch of the foot. Progressive tightening of the structure, usually in association with a tight tendo-Achilles, appears to be the prime factor in its occurrence. Again, slow stretching of this structure and the tendo-Achilles is probably the best preventor. Well-cushioned, stable running shoes are also important, as is slow, progressive training.

It must be evident from this catalogue of injuries that ways to prevent certain of these problems are just beginning to be understood, but proper training, done with slow progression, is the most important step in preventing their occurrence, despite the great variety of tissue involved. Since the recreational athletes are frequently their own coaches, there is truly no one to blame but the self for failure to avoid these injuries.

References

1. Brubaker, C.E., and James, S.L. Injuries to runners. *Am. J. Sports Med.* 2:189–198, 1974.

2. Buxbaum, R., and Micheli, L.J. *Sports for Life.* Boston: Beacon Press, 1979.

3. Clarke, K.S. Premises and pitfalls of athletic injury surveillance. *J. Sports Med.* 3:292–295, 1975.

4. Drez, D. Running footwear. *Am. J. Sports Med.* 8:140–141, 1980.

5. Guten, G. Herniated nucleus pulposus in the runner. *Am. J. Sports Med.*, in press.

6. Micheli, L.J. Sports injuries in children and adolescents. In R.H. Strauss (Ed.), *Sports Medicine and Physiology.* Philadelphia, Penn.: W.B. Saunders Co., 1979.

7. Micheli, L.J. Female runners. In R.D. D'Ambrosia (Ed.), *Prevention and Treatment of Running Injuries.* Charles B. Slack, 1980.

8. Micheli, L.J., Santopietro, F.J., Gerbino, P.G., et al. Etiologic assessment of overuse stress fractures in athletes. *Nova Scotia Bulletin.* Pp. 43–47, April/June 1980.

9. Puddu, G. Method for reconstruction of the anterior cruciate ligament using the semitendinosus tendon. *Am. J. Sports Med.* 8(6):402–404, 1980.

10. Stanish, W.D. Treatment of chronic tendinitis with eccentric exercise training. Presented at the Am. Acad. Orthop. Surg. meeting, Las Vegas, Nevada, February 24, 1981.

11. Vinger, P.F., and Tolpin, D.W. Racket sports: An ocular hazard. *JAMA,* 239:2575–2577, 1978.

14 Head and Cervical Spine Injuries

Robert C. Cantu, M.D.

Introduction

The central nervous system, the brain and spinal cord, is unique in that nerve cells are incapable of regeneration. Injury to these structures takes on a singular importance as cells that die are forever lost, incapable of regrowth, transplantation, or replacement with artificial hardware. While virtually every major joint (ankle, knee, hip, elbow, shoulder) and most of the body's organs are capable of replacement, the central nervous system housed in the skull and spine is the sole organ where this is not posssible.

With these sobering facts in mind, the clinical evaluation of the head- or spine-injured athlete takes on a singular importance [1]. The clinical assessment must be expeditious, precise, and forever bearing in mind the Hippocratic prohibition: "First, do no harm."

Whenever the injury involves a loss of consciousness, several important simultaneous observations and assumptions must be made. Assume the patient has a fractured neck and carry out the examination with this in mind. First, determine the patient has an adequate airway; then conduct a rapid baseline medical and neurological examination. This should include blood pressure, pulse, respiratory rate, state of consciousness (alert, stupor, semicomatose, comatose), pupillary size and reactivity, extremity movement spontaneously and in response to painful stimulation, deep tendon and Babinski reflexes.

This initial examination is crucial to subsequent evaluation and treatment. If the patient shows improvement within a few minutes, then subsequent transportation and diagnostic evaluation can proceed in a routine manner. If, however, deterioration, especially in the state of consciousness, is seen, then transportation and subsequent treatment must be precipitous. Every unconscious athlete should be transported on a fracture board. The head should be secured in a neutral position with sand bags, four-poster collar, or traction device if available.

If the unconscious athlete is wearing a helmet and has a good airway, do not remove the helmet as this may precipitate a quadriplegia if an unstable cervical fracture is present. Only if the airway is questionable, should the helmet be removed, and then never forcibly and always with the neck in a neutral (neither flexed nor extended) position. The helmet can be used for cervical traction. The chin strap serves as the halter and the ear holes and/or immediately adjacent edge of the helmet as a site for attachment of neutral traction. While the unconscious athlete is being moved onto the spine board, the ear holes of the helmet also may serve as a convenient site to insert one's index finger to effect gentle neutral cervical traction. Only after appropriate cervical spine x-rays have excluded a cervical spine fracture, malalignment, or instability can the helmet be safely removed from the unconscious athlete.

In the event that a fracture board is not readily available to transport the unconscious athlete from the site of injury, a decision must be made whether to wait for the ambulance to arrive with its stretcher or transport the athlete using the locked-arm technique. While one might generally favor the former, it is true that if adequate players or spectators are present, by locking hands to elbows of individuals standing opposite each other, a secure surface for transporting an injured athlete a short distance is provided. When transporting an unconscious athlete in this manner, one person applies neutral traction to the helmet or otherwise secures the head in a neutral position.

Sports Most Hazardous to the Head and Cervical Spine

Sports of maximal risk to the head and cervical spine are automobile racing, diving, football (only team sport), hang gliding, and motorcycle racing. Sports with high risk for the head and cervical spine injury are gymnastics, horseback riding, mountain climbing, parachuting, ski jumping, sky diving, sky gliding, snowmobiling, and trampolining. One study of automobile racing showed that during their initial two years 30% of new participants were either killed or so seriously injured that they could not compete again [1]. Motor- (or as one might prefer sui-) cycles are even more dangerous. Eighty percent of the serious injuries befall those riding six months or less. Hang gliding ranks at the top in terms of fatalities or serious injury per participant. Amazingly, the use of adequate helmets is not even uniformly seen in this sport.

The mechanism of cervical spine injury is illustrated in figures 14-1 and 14-2. In neutral posture, the neck has a gentle S-shaped curve (figure 14-1). When the neck is flexed (figure 14-2), the spine becomes straight. With the vertebral bodies lined up straight, vertical impact forces are directly transmitted from one vertebra to the next, allowing for minimal dissipation of the impact forces to be absorbed by the muscles. If the impact force exceeds the strength of the bone, it compacts it at one or more levels causing a compression fracture. If the fractured vertebra malaligns and is driven back into the spinal cord, quadriplegia may result. Table 14–1 shows the mechanism of injury in football permanent cervical quadriplegia.

It is when tackling with the head (see table 14–2), especially in the open field where momentum is greatest, that most serious neck injuries occur [6]. The small defensive back is most susceptible (table 14–3). The fast but light safety is injured attempting to bring down a larger, heavier back with a head tackle. The high school athlete, where the degree of physical maturation and athletic ability has the greatest degree of variation, is at greatest risk (see tables 14–4 and 14–5).

At present, catastrophic football head and neck injuries are at the lowest level in the last eighteen years, approximately 0.5 per 100,000 athletes [3]. This represents an over 600% reduction from peak years in the later 1960s and directly reflects the 1976 rule change to prohibit butt blocking and face tackling. It also stems from the football helmet standard established by the National Operating Committee on Standards for Athletic Equipment, improved conditioning programs, and improved supervision by team physicians and trainers.

While football fatalities and catastrophic injuries will never be totally eliminated, their occurrence is now rare. Most entire football conferences go decades without such a problem, while yearly almost each participating school has one or more fatalities or catastrophic injuries attributed to a car or motorcycle accident. For the high school student, it is clearly more dangerous to drive a car or motorcycle than to play football.

Table 14–1
Football Permanent Cervical Quadriplegia, 1971–1975

Mechanism of Injury	Number of Injuries
Hyperflexion	10
Hyperextension	3
Vertical compression (spearing)	52
Knee/thigh to head	15
Collision/pile/ground contact	11
Tackled	7
Machine-related	3
Face-mask acting as lever	0

Source: Reproduced with permission from the book *Health Maintenance through Physical Conditioning* edited by Robert C. Cantu ©1981 by PSG Publishing Company.

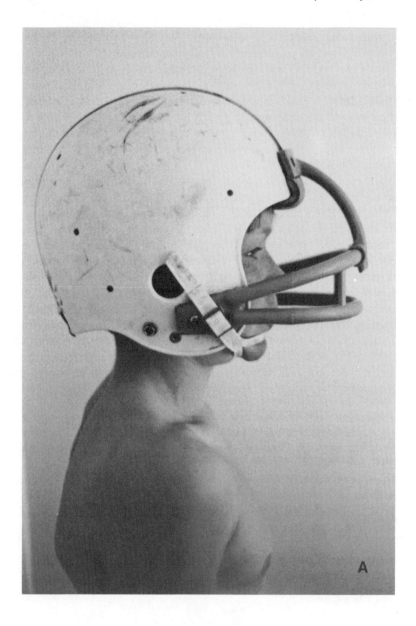

Figure 14–1. A and B. Normal Neutral Neck Posture. Reproduced with permission from *Health Maintenance through Physical Conditioning* edited by Robert C. Cantu. Copyright ©1981 by PSG Publishing Company.

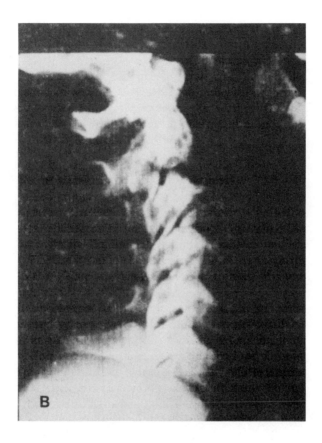

Cranial Athletic Injuries

Concussion

Far and away the most common athletic brain injury is a concussion. While physiologically defined as a transient alteration of brain function (usually with a period of unconsciousness) and then complete brain recovery, many a concussion occurs without a lapse in consciousness. This has led to a clinical grading of concussion in which in the most mild form, grade I, there is no loss of consciousness but only lapse of memory after the head trauma. Many a boxer has instinctively gone on to win a fight after a blow to the head that rendered him amnesic for events after an early round. It is not uncommon for a football player to have his bell rung during a given play and then continue playing the rest of the game without subsequent recall.

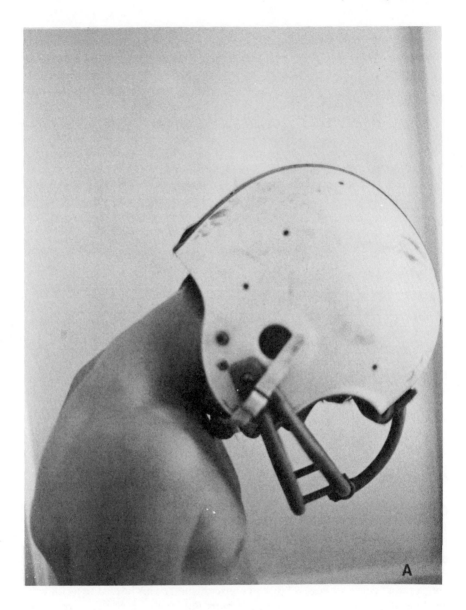

Figure 14-2. A and B. Flexed Spearing Neck Posture. Reproduced with permission from *Health Maintenance through Physical Conditioning* edited by Robert C. Cantu. Copyright ©1981 by PSG Publishing Company.

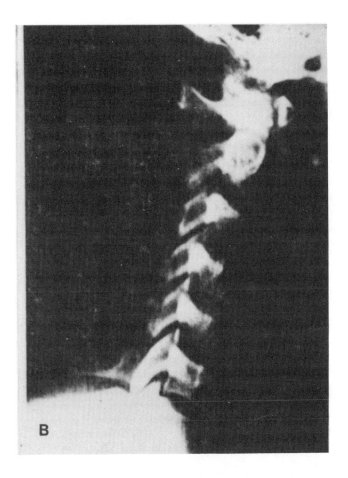

B

In the more severe grades of concussion, one is unconscious transiently (grade II) or for a more prolonged time (grade III). In this instance, the head trauma causes alterations in the function of the reticular activating system which runs from the upper-cervical spinal cord to the thalamus. This results in unconsciousness and associated changes in pulse, respiration, and blood pressure. As the reticular activating system resumes normal function, consciousness, motor power, and coordination are regained.

Generally speaking, the degree and duration of amnesia correlates with the severity of the concussion. In grade I, the amnesia is usually only for events immediately after the head trauma (retrograde amnesia). However, in grade III, events preceding the trauma may also be lost (antegrade amnesia). For the schoolboy athlete, a grade II or III concussion (a period of unconsciousness) mandates removal from the game, obtaining skull x-rays, and placement in a medical facility for 24 hours of neurological observation. With a grade I concussion in certain instances where the player

Table 14-2
Football Injury by Activity, 1971–1975

	Permanent Cervical Quadriplegia (%)	
	High School	College
Tackling	72	78
Tackled	14	22
Blocking	6	0
Drill	3	0
Collision/pile-up	3	0
Machine-related	2	0

Source: Reproduced with permission from the book *Health Maintenance through Physical Conditioning* edited by Robert C. Cantu ©1981 by PSG Publishing Company.

Table 14-3
Football Injuries by Position, 1971–1975

	Permanent Cervical Quadriplegia (%)	
	High School	College
Defensive back	52	73
Linebacker	10	0
Specialty team	13	7
Offensive back	11	7
Defensive line	10	0
Offensive line	4	13

Source: Reproduced with permission from the book *Health Maintenance through Physical Conditioning* edited by Robert C. Cantu ©1981 by PSG Publishing Company.

is fully lucid with no headache, return to play is permissible. However, that player should be observed closely over the next 24 hours in case an expanding intracranial mass (blood clot) is developing. The player should be awakened every two hours during the night and under no circumstance allowed to be left alone that first night.

Occasionally the head trauma wil be sufficient to produce a degree of brain swelling (edema) over the ensuing 24 hours. This may result in headache. An athlete should be free of headache at rest before resuming the

Table 14-4
Football Cervical Spine Fracture-Dislocations, 1971-1975

	Number of Injuries
High School	182
College	64
Other	13
Total	259

Source: Reproduced with permission from the book *Health Maintenance through Physical Conditioning* edited by Robert C. Cantu ©1981 by PSG Publishing Company.

Table 14-5
Football Permanent Quadriplegias, 1971-1975

	Number of Injuries
High School	77
College	18
Other	4
Total	99

Source: Reproduced with permission from the book *Health Maintenance through Physical Conditioning* edited by Robert C. Cantu ©1981 by PSG Publishing Company.

sport, and free of headache at maximal intensity training before returning to competition.

The question of allowing an athlete to return to competition after repeated concussions is still controversial. For the nonprofessional student-athlete, it is generally agreed that two concussions of grade II or III severity during any one season should exclude that athlete from further participation that season.

When the athlete is free of headache at maximal exertion and has a normal electroencephalogram, that athlete may safely resume competition after a first concussion. However, before this is allowed, a thorough review of the circumstances resulting in the concussion should be effected. If available, videotapes or game films should be reviewed by the player, coach, and trainer. It should be determined if the player was using the head unwisely, illegally, or both. This review will also reveal if the player is wearing the equipment correctly. Finally, the equipment itself should be rechecked to be certain it not only is worn properly but fits correctly as well.

Intracranial Hemorrhage

The leading cause of death from athletic head injury is intracranial hemorrhage. There are four types of hemorrhage to which the examining trainer or physician must be alert in every instance of head injury. Since all four types of intracranial hemorrhage may be fatal, both rapid, accurate initial assessment as well as appropriate follow-up is mandatory after an athletic head injury.

An epi- or extradural hematoma is usually the most rapidly progressing intracranial hematoma. It is frequently associated with a fracture in the temporal bone and results from a tear in one of the arteries supplying the covering (dura) of the brain. The hematoma accumulates inside the skull but outside the covering of the brain. Arising from a torn artery, it may progress quite rapidly and reach a fatal size in 30 to 60 minutes. Although not always present, the athlete may have a lucid interval; that is, initially the athlete may regain consciousness after the head trauma, before starting to experience increasing headache and progressive deterioration in level of consciousness as the clot accumulates and the intracranial pressure increases. This lesion, if present, will almost always declare itself within an hour or two from the time of injury. Usually the brain substance is free from direct injury; thus, if the clot is promptly removed surgically, a full recovery is to be expected. Because this lesion is rapidly and universally fatal if missed, all athletes receiving a head injury must be very closely and frequently observed during the ensuing several hours, preferably the next 24 hours. This observation should be effected where full neurosurgical services are immediately available.

A subdural hematoma, a second type of intracranial hemorrhage, occurs between the brain surface and the dura. It is, thus, under the dura and directly on the brain. It often results from a torn vein running from the surface of the brain to the dura. It may also result from a torn venous sinus or even a small artery on the surface of the brain. With this injury, there is often associated injury to the brain tissue. If a subdural hematoma necessitates surgery in the first 24 hours, the mortality is high not due to the clot itself but to the associated brain damage. With a subdural hematoma that progresses rapidly, the athlete usually does not regain consciousness and immediate neurosurgical evaluation is obvious. Occasionally, the brain itself will not be injured, and a subdural hematoma may slowly develop over a period of days to weeks. This chronic subdural hematoma, although often associated with headache, may initially present a variety of very mild, almost imperceptible mental, motor, or sensory signs and symptoms. Since its recognition and removal will lead to full recovery, it must always be suspected in an athlete who has previously sustained a head injury and who days or weeks later is not quite right. A CAT scan of the head will definitively show such a lesion.

An intracerebral hematoma is the third type of intracranial hemorrhage seen after head trauma. In this instance, the bleeding is into the brain substance itself, usually from a torn artery. It may also result from the rupture of a congenital vascular lesion such as an aneurysm or arteriovenous malformation. Intracerebral hematomas are not usually associated with a lucid interval and may be rapidly progressive. Death occasionally occurs before the injured athlete can be moved to a hospital. Because of the intense reaction such a tragic event precipitates among fellow athletes, family, students, and even the community at large and because of the inevitable rumors that follow, it is imperative to obtain a complete autopsy in such an event to clarify fully the causative factors. Often the autopsy will reveal a congenital lesion that may indicate the cause of death was other than presumed and ultimately unavoidable. Only by such full, factual elucidation will inappropriate feelings of guilt in fellow athletes, friends, and family be assuaged.

A fourth type of intracranial hemorrhage is subarachnoid or confined to the surface of the brain. Following head trauma, such bleeding is the result of disruption of the tiny surface brain vessels and is analogous to a bruise. Like the intracerebral hematoma, there is often brain swelling, and such a hemorrhage can also result from a ruptured cerebral aneurysm or arteriovenous malformation. In that bleeding is superficial, surgery is not usually required unless a congenital vascular anomaly is present.

Such a contusion of the brain usually causes headache and not infrequently associated neurological deficit, depending on the area of the brain involved. The irritative properties of the blood may also precipitate a seizure. If a seizure occurs in a head-injured athlete, it is important to log-roll the patient onto his side. By this maneuver, any blood or saliva will roll out of the mouth or nose, and the tongue cannot fall back obstructing the airway. If one has a padded tongue depressor or oral airway, it can be inserted between the teeth. Under no circumstances should one insert their fingers into the mouth of an athlete who is having a seizure as a traumatic amputation can easily result from such an unwise maneuver. Usually such a traumatic seizure will last only for a minute or two. The athlete will then relax, and transportation to the nearest medical facility can be effected.

Cervical Spine Athletic Injuries

The same traumatic lesions just discussed for the brain may also occur to the cervical spinal cord, that is, concussion, contusion, and the various types of hemorrhage. As previously detailed in the introduction, the major concern with a cervical spine injury is the possibility of an unstable fracture that may produce quadriplegia. At the time of injury, there is no way to determine the presence of an unstable fracture until appropriate x-rays are taken. There is also no way of determining a fully recoverable from a permanent case of quadriplegia. If the patient is fully conscious, the presence of a cervical fracture or cervical cord injury is usually accompanied by rigid cervical muscle spasm and pain that immediately alerts the athlete and physician to the presence of such an injury. It is the unconscious athlete, who is unable to state that the neck hurts and whose neck muscles are not in protective spasm, that is susceptible to potential cord severence if one does not always think of the possibility of an unstable cervical spine fracture. It is imperative with an unconscious or obviously neck-injured athlete that no neck manipulation be carried out on the field. Definitive treatment must await appropriate x-rays at a medical facility, and all the precautions discussed previously must be carried out.

In addition to the aforementioned neck injuries, other lesions include a stretch or traction injury to the brachial plexus or a nerve root. This condition, termed a burner by athletes, usually results from a forceful blow to the head from the side but can result also from head extension or by depression of the shoulder while the head and neck are fixed. The athlete experiences a shocklike sensation of pain and numbness radiating into the arm and hand. Repeated injury of this type over a period of years may lead to weakness of the deltoid, biceps, and teres major muscles as well as constant pain. The use of a high cervical collar, which limits lateral neck flexion and extension, changing the athlete's hitting technique, or moving the athlete to another position may eliminate the problem. If it repeatedly recurs, however, it is suggested the athlete cease playing football or whatever the responsible contact sport and move to another athletic pursuit.

If the athlete sustains burnerlike symptoms but the pain, numbness, or weakness persists, usually with neck pain and spasm, a ruptured cervical disc is to be suspected. Such a lesion often exists in a young athlete without any abnormality on routine cervical spine x-rays.

A final uncommon but very serious neck injury involves the carotid arteries. By either extremes of lateral flexion or extension or a forceful blow by a relatively fixed narrow object such as a stiffened forearm or a cross-country ski tip impaling one's neck in a forward fall, the inner layer (intima) of the carotid may be torn. This can lead to clot formation at the site of injury resulting in emboli to the brain or more commonly a complete occlusion of the artery, causing a major stroke.

It is recommended that an athlete not return to competition after a neck injury until the athlete is free of any neck or arm pain at rest and has a full range of neck motion without discomfort or spasm. Rockett has described further criteria used at Harvard University [4]. Each athlete is measured as to the maximum weight that athlete can pull with the neck in flexion, extension, and to each side. This becomes the neck profile. Athletes with neck injuries are not allowed to return to competition until they can perform to the level of their neck profiles.

Prevention of Cervical Spine Athletic Injuries

The prevention of athletic head injuries is largely limited to using appropriate protective headgear such as the National Operating Committee on Standards for Athletic Equipment's football helmet and then taking one's chances. The brain cannot be preconditioned to accept trauma: rather the reverse is true. That is, once the brain is injured, it is more susceptible to future injury.

Quite in contrast to the brain, the neck can be strengthened, and the risk of injury reduced. Nautilus machines are now available that strengthen the neck in all four movements: flexion, extension, lateral bending, and rotation. These same exercises can be carried out without machines using the resistance of a fellow colleague's wrist. While controversy exists as to whether the neck can be conditioned to withstand the maximum forces to which it may be subjected in contact sports, a neck exercise program, as suggested by the National Football League Management Council [2], is universally agreed to minimize the risk of neck injury.

Finally, since most serious neck injuries occur in diving accidents, almost all in unsupervised recreation, the following tips from Shields et al. [5] bear repeating:

1. Never dive into unfamiliar water.

2. Do not assume the water is deep enough. Even familiar lakes, rivers, and swimming holes change levels.

3. If you are present at a spinal cord injury, keep the victim's head and neck from bending and twisting.

4. Never dive near dredging or construction work. The water level may have dropped and dangerous objects may be just beneath the surface.

5. Do not drink before diving or swimming. Alcohol distorts judgment.

6. Water around a raft can be dangerous, especially if the water level is down. A slackened cable permits the raft to drift, putting the cable and anchor into the diving area.

7. Cloudy water can conceal hazardous objects. Check the bottom.

Thus, when the sport is intelligently pursued with adequate protection and preparation, the athlete can play a variety of potentially hazardous sports with little risk of injury. There is no substitute for the faithful daily execution of an appropriate exercise program, and the head must never be employed as a battering ram. The ultimate responsibility for avoiding head and spine injuries lies with the athletes themselves and the physicians, coaches, and trainers who advise them.

References

1. Bodnar, L.M. Sports medicine with reference to back and neck injuries. *Curr. Pract. Orthop. Surg.* 7:116–153, 1977.

2. Cushing, D. NFL expands roughness rules. *Phys. Sports Med.* 7:17–18, 1979.

3. Mueller, F.O., and Blyth, C.S. Catastrophic head and neck injuries. *Phys. Sports Med.* 7:71–74, 1979.

4. Rockett, F.X. Injuries involving the head and neck: Clinical and anatomic aspects. In P.F. Vinger and E.F. Hoerner (Eds.), *Sports Injuries: the Unthwarted Epidemic.* Littleton, Mass.: PSG Publishing Co., 1981.

5. Shields, C.L., Jr., Fox, J.M., and Stauffer, E.S. Cervical cord injuries in sports. *Phys. Sports Med.* 6:71–76, 1978.

6. Torg, J.S., Quedenfeld, T.C., Burstein, A., et al. National football head and neck injury registry: Report on cervical quadriplegia. *Am. J. Sports Med.* 7:127–132, 1979.

15   Lumbar Spine Injuries

Robert C. Cantu, M.D.

Low back pain is a very common ailment in the athlete and nonathlete alike [1,5]. It is the second most common medical symptom—the first is headache—and runner-up only to the common cold in days missed from work; today it is a major health problem with over $15 billion expended annually on its treatment and compensation [4]. In fact, compensation for low back disorders in industry represents an amount exceeding that of all other injuries combined [2].

What are the causes of low back pain? Why are young, vigorous, physically fit, elite male and female athletes suffering the same symptoms so prevalent in the unfit, sedentary middle-aged? The answers to these questions and the elimination of the problem require an understanding of the anatomy and pathology of low back pain.

Five mobile lumbar vertebrae with cartilaginous cushions (discs) between them and the fused bones of the sacrum and coccyx, which form the back of the pelvis, compose the lower back. Ligaments (thick, dense, tough strands of connective tissue) hold the foundation blocks of the low back, the vertebrae, sacrum, coccyx, and pelvis together. All these ligaments have some elasticity and thus provide the back with mobility. The five major groups of low back ligaments and their mechanism of injury include:

Annulus fibrosus. This is the hard, outer circumferential covering of the nucleus pulposus or disc. The radial relationship of the fibers adds strength and has been copied by industry with the radial-ply tire. The annuli serve to restrict excessive motion between the vertebrae and to hold in place the nuclei pulposi (discs) with their resultant cushion effect.

Anterior and posterior longitudinal ligaments. These run front (anterior) and back (posterior) along the longitudinal surface from one vertebra to another. They blend with and reinforce the annuli fibrosi. The anterior is much stronger than the posterior; the posterior disc ruptures more often than the anterior.

Ligamenta flava. These form the roof of the spinal canal and bind rear segments of vertebrae. They are more elastic than other ligaments and are rarely torn.

Some of the text in this chapter is reproduced with permission from *Health Maintenance through Physical Conditioning* edited by Robert C. Cantu © 1981 by PSG Publishing Company.

Interspinal ligaments. These ligaments extend from one spinous process to another and limit forward bending. They relax in extension and are torn or ruptured by extremes of forward bending motion (flexion).

Intertransverse ligaments. These ligaments extend from one transverse process to another and limit sideward bending. They are torn or ruptured by extremes of sideward bending.

The muscles of the back, abdomen, and hip are responsible for both support and movement of the back. There are four groups of muscles essential for support of the back that can play a major role in back pain. It is convenient to think of the low back as a pole held erect by four guy-wire muscle groups: the abdominal, the extensor, and the two sides.

Abdominal muscles. These anterior guy wires are the rectus abdominus, internal oblique, external oblique, and transverse abdominus muscles. They extend from the rib cage to the sides and front of the pelvis where they attach by strong, rough connective tissues called tendons. They support the abdominal cavity and control bending movements of the spine. When they are tensed, they relieve strain on the back. Investigators have demonstrated that it is the strong abdominal muscles that allow one to lift weights that would otherwise crush the spine.

Extensor muscles. These posterior guy wires consist of many layers, some spanning a single vertebra and others many, from the low back to the neck. Their tendons attach to the spine, pelvis, ribs, and head. These muscles are maximally used for pulling or pushing a heavy object. They are injured by posterior (arching) movements of the back.

Side muscles. The two lateral guy-wire groups control the sideward bending of the back by contraction of the quadratus lumborum and the psoas major. The psoas major is one of the body's largest muscles running from the side of the spine through the pelvis to attach to the anterior surface of the femur just below the hip joint.

These three groups of muscles, the abdominal, extensor, and two side muscles, constitute the four guy wires to support the back. However, the hips, by virtue of their relationship to the pelvis and thus the pelvis to the spine, can have a very significant effect on the back. Of the four muscle groups, the flexors (lift hips up), abductors (turn hips out), adductors (turn hips in), and extensors (lift hips back), the latter are the most massive and important to the back. The hip extensor muscles as a group control lumbar lordosis, a condition that when excessive is called sway back by the layperson and is a major cause of back pain. The hip extensors in combination with the hip flexors are essential in the maintenance of good posture.

Common Causes of Low Back Pain in the Athlete

Less than 5% of athletic back injuries involve a ruptured disc or spine fracture. The definitive medical treatment of these disorders is beyond the scope of this book, but their early recognition and emergency care is vital and will be covered later.

Almost all athletic injuries to the low back involve either a contusion, a bruise from a direct blow; a sprain, a pulling with stretching and tearing of the muscles or their tendons; or a strain, a tearing of a ligament. In general, a strain is most painful when the back is forced in the opposite direction, and a sprain produces pain when the affected muscle is contracted. From a practical standpoint due to the intricate relationships of the muscles, tendons, and ligaments of the back and the fact that most injuries involve two or all three entities, trying to separate them is academic.

The cause of most back strains and sprains in the athlete and nonathlete alike is weak muscles, especially the abdominal muscles and hip flexors, and tension or lack of flexibility, especially in the hamstring hip extensor muscles. How could world-class athletes have weak muscles? This occurs because during intensive training for the specific requirements of their sport, they neglect anatomic areas (the back-abdomen-hip) that do not seem to require development for success in their sport. At the 1976 Olympics, the Canadian medical team found the abdominal muscles underdeveloped in many world-class athletes [5]. Some of Canada's top athletes had trouble executing more than one or two bent-knee sit-ups. In general, athletes have strong extensor muscles (the back and hip), and the flexor muscles in one or both regions are frequently underdeveloped.

Mechanisms of Back Strain and Sprain

Most strains and sprains develop in one of two ways. The first is by a sudden, abrupt, violent extension contraction on an overloaded, unprepared, or underdeveloped spine, especially when there is some rotation in the attempted movement. This can result in stretching a few fibers, a complete tear, or an avulsion fracture of a spinous or transverse process.

The second mechanism involves a chronic strain, often with associated poor posture—excessive lumbar lordosis. Here there is a continuation of the underlying disease with recurring injury to the original and/or adjacent sites.

Through the repetition of training, many sports predispose one to low back pain. Most sports involve either strong back extension movements, as opposed to strong flexion, or else external forces that produce extension. Track athletes run in forced extension. The discus thrower, shot putter, and weight lifter all propel heavy weights with the back extended. Gymnasts repeatedly dismount with a hyperextended low back as the feet hit the mat. So, too, the diver hits the water in extension with foot-entry dives.

Examination of Back Injuries

Acute

For practical purposes, the back examination of an acutely injured athlete seen on the athletic field will be discussed separately from the ambulatory back-injured patient seen in the office or clinic. The essential medical equipment for this examination includes your hands, a pin, and a reflex hammer. Ice or ethylene chloride freezing spray and a fracture board or rigid stretcher represent the primary on-the-field treatment aids.

When an athlete is stricken with a back injury during competition, whether it is after a tackle in football, a slide in baseball, a fall in basketball, or riding the pole back down to the ground as happened to one high school jumper who froze with the pole in his hands, the initial examination should be on the spot. Although unstable fractures and fracture-dislocations with and without neurologic involvement are uncommon in the low back, a careful examination to eliminate their presence is essential as suspicion alone dictates great care in transport. When one arrives at the side of the conscious injured athlete, the first question asked is where does it hurt? For the back-injured athlete, even before examining the back, the next question is whether any loss of feeling or numbness or weakness is appreciated in the lower extremities. The spinal cord ends at the lower border of the first lumbar vertebra in most adults. Injury to the spinal cord usually implies a fracture-dislocation or dislocation of the vertebra at the instant of impact with spontaneous relocation. Both should be considered unstable, and the athlete should be transported off the field and to a hospital on a fracture board.

Injury to the spinal cord may produce either complete or incomplete loss of function of the nervous system below the level of the lesion. In a complete lesion, sensation, motor power, and reflexes in the legs are lost as well as bowel and bladder control. In an incomplete lesion, varying degrees of these functions are retained. The seriousness of either a complete or incomplete lesion of the spinal cord renders essential a neurologic evaluation of sensation, movement, and knee and ankle reflexes as soon as the patient is seen. If any neurologic deficit is recorded, then the patient must be transported from the field on a fracture board.

Fortunately, few back injuries have neurologic impairment. Once it is determined that there is none, the back muscles themselves should be examined. Palpation of the back should start in the midline with a thumb pressing over each spinous process. Exquisite pain over one spinous process suggests a possible fracture or tear of the interspinal ligaments. Such a fracture rarely has associated vertebral instability. Pain described as deep in the back with localized tenderness either over one or in between two spinous processes raises suspicion for a compression fracture of a vertebra. Most compression fractures involve either the 11th or 12th dorsal vertebra or one of the first two lumbar vertebrae. The young pole vaulter previously mentioned who did not let go of his pole and rode it back down incurred a fracture-dislocation of the first and second lumbar vertebrae. While most compression fractures, like spinous or transverse process fractures, are stable, if suspected due to focal midline tenderness on palpation, it is wisest to transport the injured athlete on a fracture board until such time as x-rays clearly establish that the fracture is stable. The definitive treatment of these fractures and their complications from paralytic ileus to neurologic deficit to decubitus ulcers is beyond the intent of this chapter.

Now having eliminated the most worrisome back injuries as will usually be the case, continue to palpate the back paraspinal muscles; also continue around the abdominal wall being certain to include the side flexor and rotator muscles. Areas of focal tenderness may be found that indicate local spasm. If a large swelling is present, this usually represents a contusion with hemorrhage into the muscle. A slight swelling could indicate contusion, strain, sprain, or any combination thereof. The immediate treatment is application of cold to the trigger point, either by an ice pack or freezing spray. Later treatment will involve heat, rest, and analgesic and anti-inflammatory medication. In virtually all of these injuries, the athlete can safely walk from the field under his own power.

Nonacute

A small percentage of athletes with low back problems will not only have low back pain, but also pain that radiates from the back into the buttock and/or down one or both legs. Coughing, sneezing, straining to pass urine or at bowel movements usually makes the leg pain worse. Numbness may also be felt, usually in the foot either over the medial half or along the lateral side. This pattern of pain is called sciatica and suggests that a ruptured disc is pressing on a nerve root. Discs are the fibrocartilaginous cushions between the vertebrae. As the body ages, the discs lose fluid content, becoming slightly narrower and causing a slight shrinkage in height. The outer more fibrous capsule of the disc, called the annulus fibrosus, may also tear, allowing the disc to rupture posteriorly out of the disc space and compress the nerve root as it exits from the spine. Most simple ruptures can be treated successfully with a period of bedrest, muscle relaxants, anti-inflammatory medicines, analgesics, and later, exercises. A minor percentage with neurologic deficit, that is, a reflex absence at knee or ankle, weakness of ankle or great toe extension, or persistent pain and numbness, will require surgical excision of the ruptured disc. With careful selection, the success of such surgery should exceed 90%. Following surgery, the athlete should adhere to the exercises and advice given in this chapter and should be able to resume competition.

A third group of athletes with low back problems suffer from mechanical malalignment of the vertebrae—spondylolisthesis. This diagnosis is established by x-ray of the back. If there is instability documented by further malalignment as the back is placed through flexion and extension maneuvers, then a surgical procedure of lumbar fusion may be indicated [6,7]. An abnormal lateral curvature of the spine (scoliosis) is yet another cause of low back pain. If severe in children, this may require surgical correction that is a very extensive and time-consuming procedure. Severe scoliosis renders athletic excellence very remote. The mild form seen in some athletes can be pain-free if the exercises and hints in this chapter are followed. Only a physician, and especially an orthopedist or neurosurgeon, is properly qualified to evaluate and treat the athlete's low back problem. Thus, the exercises and advice in this chapter are primarily directed at the athlete with low back pain but without neurologic deficit or one who has already had concern for a ruptured disc or spinal instability eliminated by appropriate medical consultation.

The vast majority of athletes with low back pain will have no neurologic symptoms, deficits, or spinal instability. Palpation, as with the acute injury of the paraspinal, side flexor and rotator, and abdominal muscles, usually reveals segmental spasm, tenderness, or an area of point tenderness.

Athletes are usually thin, quite physically fit, but have an accentuated lumbar lordosis when walking. The posterior erector spinal muscles are strong, but the abdominal (flexor) muscles, although flat, in comparison are quite weak. A good test of abdominal muscle strength is a slow bent-knee sit-up. An athlete should be able to do 20 or more, but some Olympic-class athletes with back problems have trouble doing one [5]. The back extensor muscles are tested with the athlete on his abdomen with a pillow under the hips as a cushion. To test the upper back, with the hands behind the head, raise elbows, chin, and trunk off the floor as long as possible. Low back strength is tested by keeping the head down with hands behind while both legs held together with knees straight are raised off the floor. In both exercises, 20 seconds indicates strong muscles and under 10 weak.

Frequently, back rotation is weak. When the overdeveloped extensors are tight, both flexion and rotation are compromised. In some athletes, the hip flexor and hamstring muscles will be tight. In such cases, one cannot touch the floor with fingertips with the knees straight. Ideally, the hamstring muscles should be at least 60% to 80% as strong as the quadriceps; the closer to 80%, the fewer back problems encountered. To test the strength of the hip flexor muscles, have the athletes lie on their backs, legs extended, hands clasped behind the head. With legs touching, have them lift their feet about ten inches off the floor and hold this position for as long as possible. Over 20 seconds indicates strong muscles, under 10 quite weak hip flexor muscles.

Treatment

The successful treatment of low back pain in athletes involves a three-step program. First is the relief of pain and spasm; second, the adoption of an appropriate exercise program that includes both stretching and strengthening exercises; third, an educational program that takes into consideration one's training program and is tailored to preventing future injuries.

Relief of Pain and Spasm

Ice, analgesics, muscle relaxants, anti-inflammatory agents, and rest are used in the acute stages while heat, muscle stimulation, and/or ultrasound, physical therapy, and the same pharmacologic agents are used 12 or more hours after injury. Ultrasound and gentle muscle stimulation seem to more rapidly dissipate muscle spasm, point tenderness, and general soreness. This is probably due to enhanced muscle circulation and exchange at the cellular level of prescribed pharmacologic agents plus elimination of toxic cellular products [3]. Actually, while modes of pain relief exist, no one treatment has been clearly demonstrated to accelerate actual tissue healing.

Stretching and Strengthening Exercises

Medications, manipulations, massage, ultrasound, and hot and cold applications do not strengthen a weakened or compromised part of the body. Low back pain is usually due to muscles that are weak, tense, fatigued, or all three. Once the healing process has occurred, it is essential to embark on an exercise program to rebuild the back and abdominal musculature. Before the strengthening exercises are commenced, it is important first to have executed specific stretching exercises for the lumbar extensor and pelvic rotator, hip flexor, and hamstring and hip extensor muscles.

Stretching. Athletes can stretch their lower-back muscles by lying on a mat and bringing the feet up over the face to touch extended toes beyond the head. It is important that these movements are executed fluidly with no sudden jerking. A good exercise to stretch the hip flexor muscles is to lie on one's back, knees bent, feet under the buttocks. When the arms reach as far toward the knees as possible, the back arches and the hips are thus maximally extended. The straight leg raise and standing with one leg on waist-high table, nose-toe touch are good flexibility exercises for the hamstrings, while the single knee raise and double knee hug stretch the hamstrings, low back, and hip extensors. The athlete must work daily on flexibility exercises to maintain a good range of motion. They should become a routine part of his daily warm-up and cool-off exercises.

Strengthening. Exercises that strengthen the low back and abdominal muscles include some of the same exercises that stretch the hamstring and hip flexor muscles. Ten such exercises will now be presented. The exercises should be carried out on a hard, flat surface with adequate padding. A tumbling mat is ideal, but a thick rug with underpadding may suffice. For those exercises done supine, most find a small pillow placed under the neck will provide more comfort. One should wear loose, unrestrictive clothing. As mentioned previously, the exercises must always be initiated slowly to allow muscles to loosen up gradually. At no time employ jerking or snapping movements. Most find that relaxing before exercising is beneficial and that heat treatment to the low back aids in loosening tight muscles. Slight discomfort may occur as the exercises are performed, but if frank pain is experienced, the exercise period should be terminated. The exercises should be done daily, ideally twice a day in the beginning. Athletes should progress at their own individual pace. Initially, five repetitions usually will suffice; then one can add a repetition or two daily to each exercise that can be accomplished with relative ease. If one or more of the exercises results in appreciable discomfort, then it should be abandoned while the remainder are continued. Only resume an exercise when it can be done without discomfort.

1. The back flattener is to strengthen gluteal (buttock) and abdominal muscles and flatten the low back in lumbar lordosis. Lie on back on padded floor with knees well bent. Relax with arms above head. A small pillow may be placed under head if desired. Squeeze buttocks together as if trying to hold a piece of paper between them. At the same time, suck in and tighten the muscles of the abdomen. The back should flatten against the floor. This is the flat back position. Hold this position for a count of ten (ten seconds), relax and repeat the exercise three times in the beginning. Gradually attempt to increase to 20 repetitions.

After the basic exercise has been done for a week or more, additional flattening can be achieved by doing the exercise with the buttocks slightly raised (one to two inches) off the floor at the time the buttocks are squeezed and abdomen tensed. Hold for the count of ten, relax, and repeat.

After several weeks of the basic exercise, gradually do the exercise with the knees less and less bent, until the exercise is executed with legs straight. The buttock raise need not be combined with this modification.

2. The single knee raise stretches low back, hip flexor, and hamstring (posterior thigh) muscles. Lie on back on a padded floor with arms above head and knees bent. Tighten buttocks and abdominal muscles as in exercise number one. Then raise one knee over chest toward chin as far as possible, hold for ten seconds, return to starting position, and relax a few seconds before repeating with the opposite leg. Start with three repetitions of each knee, gradually advancing to ten.

3. The single knee hug has the same purpose and is essentially the same exercise as the single knee raise, except the hands are not placed above the head, but rather are placed around the knee to be raised. The arms are used to pull (raise) the knee higher over the chest than was possible in exercise number two. This produces greater stretching of the low back and hamstrings. The same ten-second hold, number of repetitions, and advanced modification pertain as with the single knee raise.

4. The double knee hug stretches low back and hamstring muscles and strengthens abdominal and hip flexor muscles. Lie on back on a covered floor with knees bent, arms at sides, and pillow under the head if desired. Tighten buttocks and abdominal muscles so that low back is flat against the floor. Grasp both knees with hands and raise them slowly over chest as far as possible. Hold ten seconds, return to starting position, relax a few seconds, then repeat. Start with three repetitions and gradually build to ten.

After a month or more of the basic exercise, attempt the double knee hug starting with both legs extended straight. Tense buttocks and abdomen, and then taking care to keep the back flat, bend both knees, grasp knees with hands and raise over chest, hold ten seconds, and return to starting position to relax before repeating. The low back tends to arch when lifting and lowering the knee. If this cannot be done with the back against the floor, the athlete is not ready for this modification and should resume the basic knees-bent position. This extended-leg starting position strengthens both the hip flexing and abdominal muscles.

5. The single leg raise also stretches low back and hamstring muscles, and strengthens abdominal and hip-flexing muscles. Lie on back on a covered floor with the knee bent and one leg straight, arms at sides, and a pillow under the head if desired. Tighten buttocks and abdominal muscles, then slowly raise the straight leg, keeping it straight and the back flat. Raise the leg as far as comfortably possible, then slowly lower the leg to the floor, keeping it straight and the back flat. Relax a few seconds, and then repeat

with the other leg. Start with three repetitions of each leg, and gradually increase to ten.

After a month or more, attempt the single leg raise starting with both legs extended straight. Tense buttocks and low back and with back flat and legs out straight, raise one leg up as far as possible. As the leg is raised, back may not remain flat. Check this by using hand to see if back lifts from the floor when the leg is lifted and lowered. If it does, resume the basic exercise with one knee bent.

6. The partial sit-up strengthens low back and abdominal muscles. Lie on back on a covered floor with knees well bent. Squeeze buttocks and tighten abdominal muscles; with low back on the floor, slowly raise head, neck, and lastly shoulders while extending arms to knees. Keep low back flat on the floor. Hold this position ten seconds, return to starting position, rest a few seconds, and repeat. Start with three repetitions and progress to at least ten.

After having progressed to ten repetitions, begin progressively to lift head and shoulders farther from the floor. The back will now lift off the floor. Keep knees bent. In the beginning, it may help to place feet under a heavy chair or some other restraint. Once abdominal muscles are strong enough, this should not be necessary and not done as this action actually allows the legs to help the abdomen in raising the body. The motion should be a gentle, smooth curling and uncurling. Never jerk to achieve greater height or an additional repetition and never strain or exert beyond reasonable comfort. Again, start with three repetitions and progress to at least ten.

7. Advanced sit-up is used to maximally strengthen low back and abdominal muscles. Lie on back on a covered floor with knees well bent. Squeeze buttocks and tighten abdominal muscles. Start with arms folded over waist and lift head, shoulders, and back smoothly up to the position where arms are touching knees. Hold ten seconds, return to the starting position, relax a few seconds, and then repeat. Again, start with three repetitions and progress to at least ten.

Progress gradually until ten of the basic advanced sit-ups can be easily and comfortably executed. Then try folding the arms in front of face instead of waist. Curl up to knees, hold ten seconds, then return to the starting position, relax a few seconds, and repeat. Start with three repetitions. When this modified version can be accomplished ten times, a sit-up with hands clasped behind the head can be attempted. When this version can also be done ten times, attempt the most maximal version of a sit-up. This involves lying on the back on a padded inclined surface (that is, a tilt board with the foot end elevated). Knees should be bent as always; then with hands clasped behind neck, slowly and carefully execute the sit-up, hold ten seconds, slowly uncurl to the starting position, relax, and repeat. This last version is clearly optional. The more inclined the board, the greater strength and effort will be required of your back and abdomen to accomplish the sit-up.

8. The sitting bend strengthens the low back while stretching low back and hamstring muscles. Sit on a hard chair, feet flat on the floor, knees not more than 12 inches apart, arms folded loosely in the lap. Squeeze buttocks and tighten abdominal muscles so that back goes flat against the chair. Bend over, letting head go between knees with hands reaching for the floor. Bend as far as is comfortable, hold for a count of five, then slowly pull body back to the flatback sitting starting position. Relax a few seconds, repeat initially three times, gradually increasing to ten repetitions.

9. The deep knee bend strengthens hamstring and quadriceps muscles. Do not begin this exercise until it has been confirmed by a viewer that a good back flattener (number one) has been accomplished. Most should not attempt this exercise until a month into the exercise program. Discontinue this exercise if there is considerable lasting discomfort in your knees or hips.

Stand behind a sofa, desk, heavy chair, or similar structure holding onto it for balance. Squeeze and tighten buttocks and abdomen. Slowly bend knees and with a flat back, squat down as far as is reasonably comfortable, stop, and stand up using only legs, not arms. Relax for a second or two and repeat initially three times and gradually build up to ten repetitions.

10. Posture check helps correct standing and walking. It also determines if the exercise program is accomplishing its goals. Stand with back to the wall, pressing heels, buttocks, shoulders, and head against the wall. There should be no space between low back and the wall; if there is, the back is too arched and not flat. Move feet forward, bending knees so back slides a few inches down the wall. Now again squeeze buttocks and tighten abdominal muscles, flattening lower back against the wall. While holding this position, walk feet back so as to slide up the wall. Standing straight, walk away from the wall and around the room. Return to the wall and back up to it to be certain that the proper posture was kept.

Educational Program

The final link in the low back pain-elimination triangle involves educating the athlete in how to avoid back problems, both in training and daily life. As previously mentioned, good posture is achieved by rotating the top of the pelvis backward, which flattens the curve in the low back. Common everyday tips to avoid the occurrence of low back pain include the following:

Standing and Walking. Stand with lower back erect and as flat as possible. By squeezing buttocks and sucking in and tensing abdomen, the lower back is straightened. Walk, stand, and sit as tall as possible.

Bend knees when leaning, as when over a wash basin. Avoid leaning whenever possible and squat with a straight lower back.

Avoid high-heeled shoes. They shorten Achilles tendons and increase lordosis.

Avoid standing for long periods of time, but if it is necessary, alternate leaning on the left foot and right foot, and if possible use the bent knee position as on a stool. This flattens the lower back.

When standing, do not lean back and support body with hands. Keep hands in front of body and lean forward slightly.

When turning to walk from a standing position, move feet first and then the body.

Open doors wide enough to walk through comfortably.

Carefully judge the height of curbs before stepping up or down.

Sitting. Sit so that lower back is flat or slightly rounded outward, never with a forward curve.

Sit so that knees are higher than hips; this may require a small footstool for a short person in a high chair.

Hard seat backs that begin contact with back four to six inches above the seat and provide a flat support throughout the entire lumbar area are preferable.

Do not sit in a soft or overstuffed chair or sofa.

Avoid sitting in swivel chairs or chairs on rollers.

Do not sit with legs out straight on an ottoman or footstool.

Never sit in the same position for prolonged periods; get up and move around.

Driving. Push front seat forward so that knees will be higher than hips and the pedals are easily reached without stretching.

Sit back with back flat; do not lean forward; sit tall.

Add a flat back rest if car seat is soft or if travelling a long distance.

If on a long trip, stop every 30 to 60 minutes, get out of car and walk about, tensing buttocks and abdomen to flatten the back for several minutes.

Always fasten seatbelt and shoulder harness.

Be sure car seat has a properly adjusted headrest.

Bedrest. Sleep or rest only on a flat, firm mattress. If one is not available, place a bedboard of no less than three-quarters inch plywood under the mattress. A board of less thickness will sag, preventing proper spine alignment.

When sleeping, the preferred position is on the side, both arms in front, and knees slightly drawn up toward chin.

Do not sleep on stomach.

When lying on back, place a pillow under knees, as raising the legs flattens the lumbar curve.

When lying in bed, do not extend arms above head, relax them at sides.

If the doctor prescribes absolute bedrest, stay in bed. Raising body or twisting and turning can strain the back.

Sleep alone or in an oversized bed.

When getting out of bed, turn over on side, draw up knees, then swing legs over the side of the bed.

Lifting. When lifting, let the legs do the work, using the large muscles of the thighs instead of the small muscles of the back.

Do not twist the body; face the object.

Never lift with legs straight.

Do not lift heavy objects from car trunks.

Do not lift from a bending-forward position.

Do not reach over furniture to open and close windows.

Tuck in the buttocks and pull in the abdomen when lifting.

Only lift holding the object close to the body.

Lift a heavy load no higher than the waist and a light load no higher than the shoulders, as greater height increases lumbar lordosis.

To turn while lifting, pivot feet turning the whole body at one time.

In training, to minimize back injuries, the athlete should always warm up slowly and cool down after the main workout. Both the warm-up and cool-off periods should include back-stretching exercises. Calisthenics that involve hyperextension of the back such as back bends, straight leg sit-ups, or straight leg raises should be avoided when possible.

By faithfully carrying out a daily program of back exercises, the athlete can pursue a variety of potentially hazardous sports with minimal risk of back injury.

Sports Most Hazardous To The Back

As discussed previously, most back injuries are sustained by acute hyperextension of the back. Football is felt by some to be legalized assault, often between physical unequals. It is one of the most hazardous sports to the body and to the back in particular. This is especially true for the interior linemen (defensive ends, guards, tackles, and centers). A report from a major university with a recent number-one national ranking cited the fact that during one year, 50% of interior linemen sought medical attention for low back pain [1]. This report postulated biochemics of the back injury. As the lineman drives forward attempting to push the opponent backward, the lumbar spine is extended and this converts more of the force to a shearing force that can lead to pars interarticularis injury. It concluded that the high incidence of spondylolisthesis and spondylosis seen in interior linemen is the result of repeated forces being transmitted to the pars interarticularis while players are in the lumbar-extended posture.

Weightlifting is another high-risk back-injury sport. This is especially true for the overhead military press and the clean and jerk. Severe lordotic postures are also assumed when spiking a volleyball, hitting a twist serve or deep overhead stroke in tennis, putting the shot, throwing the discus or hammer, or even stretching for the tape in track. Extreme backward arching movements are required by the gymnast (especially in dismounts), diver, trampolinist, and squash, soccer, handball, and racquetball enthusiast. Also, sledding, downhill skiing, and snow and water-ski jumping can result in excessive stresses to the low back. Both the hang glider and pole vaulter occasionally have precipitous descents in awkward postures that can result in back strain and even compression fractures.

Sports that are less likely to result in back injury include baseball, basketball, bowling, golf, figure skating, softball, ping-pong, water skiing, canoeing, rowing, fencing, cross-country skiing, badminton, and archery. Sports least likely to result in back injury include bicycling, hiking, swimming, fishing, curling, darts, skin diving, boccie, billiards, pool, and sailing.

As emphatically repeated throughout this chapter, the athlete can best prevent low back injuries by the daily execution of appropriate muscle-stretching and strengthening exercises. For any sport, the athlete should always warm up slowly and include stretching exercises. In some sports, the most hazardous maneuvers can be modified. The serve, for example, and the overhead are the two tennis strokes most strenuous to the back. By tossing a serve slightly forward, less back extension is required and, thus, less back strain. For those who play a serve and volley game, it will also aid in gaining forward momentum toward the net. So, too, when hitting the overhead, go up to the ball hitting it slightly in front of the body. When trying for a low ball, whether tennis, handball, volleyball, softball, baseball, and so forth, whenever possible bend the knees rather than the back. Most gymnastic sports, including diving, stress good posture. The athlete at all times should sit and stand as tall as possible. The runner, equestrian, diver, and gymnast should keep the low back flat by tensing the buttocks and abdominal muscles whenever possible.

References

1. Ferguson, R.J. Low back pain in college football linemen. *J. Sports Med. Phys. Fitness* 2:63–80, 1974.

2. Friedmann, L.W., and Galton, L. *Freedom from Backaches*. New York: Pocket Books, 1973.

3. Harris, W.D. Low back pain in sports medicine. *J. Arkansas Med. Soc.* 74:377–379, 1978.

4. Nachemson, A. The lumbar spine: An orthopedic challenge. *Spine* 1:59–71, 1976.

5. Root, L., and Kiernan, T. *Oh, My Aching Back.* New York: New American Library, 1975.

6. Smith, C.F. Physical management of muscular low back pain in the athlete. *Can. Med. Assoc. J.* 177:632–635, 1977.

7. Wiltse, L.L. Etiology of spondylolisthesis. *Clin. Orthop.* 10:48–60, 1957.

8. Wiltse, L.L. Spondylolisthesis: classification and etiology. In *American Academy of Orthopedic Surgeons Symposium on the Spine.* St. Louis: C.V. Mosby, 1969.

Index

Index